Yves Dirheimer

The Craniovertebral Region in Chronic Inflammatory Rheumatic Diseases

With a Foreword by A. Wackenheim

With 86 Figures

Springer-Verlag
Berlin Heidelberg New York 1977

Docteur Yves DIRHEIMER
27, rue Goethe, F-67000 Strasbourg

ISBN-13: 978-3-642-66607-0 e-ISBN-13: 978-3-642-66605-6
DOI: 10.1007/978-3-642-66605-6

Library of Congress Cataloging in Publication Data. Dirheimer, Yves, 1934– The craniovertebral region chronic inflammatory rheumatic diseases. Includes bibliographical references and index. 1. Occipital bone – Radiography. 2. Atlas (Vertebra) – Radiography. 3. Axis (Vertebra) – Radiography. 4. Rheumatism – Diagnosis. I. Title. [DNLM: 1. Arthritis, Rheumatoid – Radiography. 2. Atlanto-occipital joint – Radiography. 3. Cervical vertebrae – Radiography. 4. Occipital bone – Radiography. 5. Joints – Pathology. WE708 D598c]. RC930.5.D57 616.7'2 77-5884

Softcover reprint of the hardcover 1st edition 1977

2123/3130 – 543210

Foreword

Radiology, the youngest of the major medical sciences, has undergone an extraordinary technical evolution since the discovery of X-rays. It began with the development of the different types of tomography and the adoption of many contrast agents, then proceeded rapidly to serioscopy, subtraction of images, direct enlargement, echography, thermography, and xerography. Today, even before all these innovations have come into common use, another branch of radiologic technology has evolved: computerized (axial) tomography. More than just an innovation, its true dimensions are unforeseeable.

Radiology has become in less than a century an indispensable adjunct to the practice of medicine. The development of radiology as a speciality followed its technical advances, which varied greatly from country to country. This rapid development led quickly to subspecialization, even the very early development of radiotherapy and radiodiagnostics as separate entities. However, the entry of radiology into the university has preserved it a single branch of medicine, avoiding the frequent tendency toward autonomy of the branches of a speciality.

Today the fourth generation of radiologists is faced with another decision: whether to become technologists subjugated to their machinery, to become subspecialists with a single skill, or to remain doctors. The vast majority of this fourth generation has rejected becoming an accessory to a master technique and rather has specialized according to the hippocratic concept of medicine.

The French school of radiology has for four decades trained neuroradiologists and radiopediatricians to be neurologists and pediatricians who are skilled in the use of radiology. Other specialities, such as vascular and gastroenterological radiology, are more difficult to delimit. Still others are so intimately involved with clinical practice that they immediately assumed an autonomous character; the borders between clinical skills per se and the radiologic aspects of the speciality have become blurred, perhaps only in theory, but still to a noteworthy degree. Senology and radiorheumatology are such subspecialities.

Doctor Yves Dirheimer pursues radiorheumatology in both the hospital and the university with a considerable degree of success. Since 1965 all of his time and energy has gone into research on the radiologic symptomatology of rheumatism. The present volume presents the results of his studies of the cervicooccipital hinge. This publication also reviews the relevant and voluminous literature from various disciplines.

As director of the radiorheumatologic team at Strasbourg, Yves Dirheimer will certainly inspire a large following. It is my wish that this work finds the place it rightfully deserves in the university of tomorrow.

Summer, 1977 A. Wackenheim

Acknowledgements

We should like to express our special thanks to Professor A. Wackenheim, head of the Department of Neuroradiology and Radiopediatry, University Hospital, Strasbourg, who for the last 10 years has been the initiator of our research on the cervicooccipital hinge. His advice has been of infinite value and he has been unfailing in encouraging us to publish this work.

Mrs. A. Wackenheim translated our manuscript into English; without her, our efforts would have remaind a rough draft in French.

For their advice and kindness in communicating certain documents to us, we should also like to thank our teachers of the Medical School of Strasbourg: A. Batzenschlager, Professor of Pathological Anatomy, F. Buchheit, Professor of Neurosurgery, E. Grosshans, Professor of Dermatology, I. Kempff, Professor of Orthopedics and Traumatology, G. Methlin, Professor of Biophysics, E. Schvingt, Professor of Orthopedics and Traumatology, H. Sick, Professor of Anatomy.

Thanks are also due to the staff members of the Department of Neuroradiology of Strasbourg, Drs. H. Ammerich, M. Haller, M. Reolon, and especially E. Babin, without forgetting the service personnel, in particular E. Bromhorst, M.R. Kipper, S. Lienhart, M. Zipfel; and E. Rittle, pathology laboratory technician.

Invaluable assistance was given to me by Drs. J.J. Ludig and P. Meyer of the radiologic service of the Clinique Bethesda, Strasbourg, who were responsible for the production of the majority of the radiographic documents and who gave us the benefit of their experience in many daily conversations. R. Anger, orthopedic surgeon, who is particularly well versed in rheumatoid arthritis surgery, also assisted us greatly.

Others who contributed to the elaboration of this publication by providing documents or making suggestions are: B. Ansell, rheumatology, Taplov; D. Baleriaux-Waha, neuroradiology, Brussels; J.P. Braun, neuroradiology, Colmar; D. Maitrot, neurosurgery, Strasbourg; J.R. Mann, pediatrics, Birmingham; O. Metzger, neurology, Strasbourg; P. Meunier, rheumatology, Lyons; G.E. Muller, neurology, Esch-sur-Alzette; L. Penning, neuroradiology, Groningen; A. Ramsheyi, general practitioner, Teheran; U. Steiger, rheumatology, Basel; W. Tempowski, radiology, Birmingham; J. Theron, neuroradiology, Caen.

Finally we must mention Dr. J. Forestier, rheumatologist and honorary president of the "Ligue Européenne contre le Rhumatisme". He has been a constant inspiration for me in my rheumatologic vocation.

May Professor W. Geinitz and all the team of Springer-Verlag, find here the expression of our gratitude for their help and understanding.

Summer, 1977 Y. Dirheimer

Contents

Material and Patients Studied

Though the author is first of all a rheumatologist, this work is mainly based on roentgenologic studies and especially on clinical experience in radiology, i.e. the documents are not simply collected from archives but concern patients who are examined and followed up clinically and biologically as well as radiologically in a rheumatologist's practice.

For instance, 345 radiological examinations have been carried out on 298 patients with chronic inflammatory rheumatisms, viz.:

	No. of patients	No. of examinations
Rheumatoid arthritis (R.A.)	174	204
Juvenile chronic polyarthritis (J.C.P.)	16	21
Ankylosing spondylitis	48	54
Psoriatic arthritis	30	33
Reiter's syndrome	7	10
Systemic lupus erythematosus	9	9
Progressive systemic sclerosis	3	3
Intestinal arthropathies	8	8
Behçet's syndrome	2	2
Sarcoidosis	1	1

As concerns rheumatoid arthritis, which will serve as a descriptive model, the number of cases studied seems to be important enough to allow some conclusions to be drawn. As concerns other diseases, we report our personal experience and the data in the literature.

The following tables provide clinical data concerning patients with rheumatoid arthritis (204 examinations in 174 patients).

Distribution with regard to the sex (174 patients)

Male:	27
Female:	147

Age of patients at time of examination (204 examinations)

20–29 years old	8
30–39 years old	28
40–49 years old	38
50–59 years old	50
60–69 years old	45
70–79 years old	32
Over 80 years old	3

Duration of evolution of rheumatoid arthritis at the time of the reported examination (204 examinations)

Less than 1 year	8
From 1 to 2 years	14
From 3 to 4 years	37
From 5 to 7 years	25
From 8 to 9 years	28
From 10 to 14 years	36
From 15 to 20 years	29
More than 20 years	27

Rheumatoid factor (174 patients)

With rheumatoid factor	149
Without rheumatoid factor	25

Rheumatoid arthritis was in all cases certain or defined according to the American Rheumatism Association criteria. Likely or possible arthritides have not been taken into account in this study.

Part 1 Historical Review

Until 20 years ago, no distinction was made between the history of an involvement of the craniovertebral joints by chronic inflammatory rheumatism and the history of spontaneous atlantoaxial subluxation. The first description of non-traumatic atlantoaxial subluxation is attributed to Sir Charles Bell, 1830 [25]. He records a patient with a deep ulcer of the pharynx who "was seized with symptoms like those of apoplexy." Two hours later "... his head fell suddenly forward, and he instantly expired." The ulcer was syphilitic and dissection led Bell to think that it had been deep enough to destroy the transverse ligament and thus to allow the dentate process of the axis "... to be thrown back so as to compress the spinal marrow." As a matter of fact, in 1931, D.M. Greig [150], Conservator of the Museum of the Royal College of Surgeons of Edinburgh, where the original specimen is still to be seen, disagreed with Bell's interpretation. He thought it more likely that the ulcer should have caused hyperemia with decalcification of the insertions of the transverse ligament and avulsion of its attachments at the level of the atlas.

In 1855, in his *Traité des Fractures et des Luxations* J.F. Malgaigne [221] distinguished different traumatic and non-traumatic etiologies. But, 17 years later, E. Bläsius, quoted by S. Werne [396], expressed the view of a solely traumatic nature of atlantoaxial dislocations, a view that will stand for several decades.

It is uncertain who first recognized atlantoaxial subluxation in rheumatoid arthritis. In 1890 A.E. Garrod [140] analyzed 500 cases of rheumatoid arthritis and pointed out the frequent involvement of the cervical spine, but he did not especially mention atlantoaxial subluxation. Toward the end of the century some authors started to consider the rheumatic nature of these changes. A. Böger [37] perhaps described the first case occurring in polyarthritis in *Ein Fall von Malum suboccipitale rheumaticum*. It seems more likely that this patient suffered from rheumatic fever; furthermore, he also had a swelling of the neck so that a local cause cannot be excluded. The case described in 1911 by L.W. Ely [115] is just as questionable. It concerns a 13-year-old child probably suffering from juvenile polyarthritis, but who also had a history of a fall while ice-skating. The traumatic nature of this case seems likely, not so much on account of the brisk onset of the troubles following the traumatism, but rather because of the extremely early stage of the polyarthritis.

In 1942 D. Englander [116] made reference to rheumatoid arthritis as a cause of occipitoatlantoaxial dislocation but did not provide any case reports. Finally, in 1951 F.W. Davis and H.E. Markley [89] actually described the first definite case of atlantoaxial subluxation in rheumatoid arthritis.

As has already been mentioned, it was at the turn of the century that the rheumatic nature of such lesions was suspected. In 1908 A. Wittek [402] reported a case of atlantoaxial subluxation following distant infection, viz. alveolar osteitis. Over the following years, several studies were published, by C.M. Jacobs, 1918 [185], P. Grisel, 1930 [151], P. Desfosses, 1930 [95], the collaborator of P. Grisel, D.M. Greig, 1931 [150], and R. Watson-Jones, 1932 [388] about spontaneous atlantoaxial dislocations occurring during or following chronic or acute infections of the base of the skull or the upper cervical region. The infections were rhinopharyngitis (P. Grisel [151]; P. Desfosses [95]; R. Watson-Jones [388]), amygdalitis (H. Swanberg [347]; P. Grisel [151]), retropharyngeal abcess (K.I. Lounavaara [216]), scarlet fever (J.H. Hess et al. [173]), mastoiditis (B. Tedesco et al. [351];

R. Watson-Jones [388]), acute articular rheumatism (C.M. Jacobs [185]; E.J. Berkheiser [27]; M.B. Coutts [81]).

The term "spontaneous" was first used by R. Watson-Jones in his report entitled "spontaneous hyperemic dislocation of the atlas." Indeed, this definition has the advantage of distinguishing traumatic cases from non-traumatic ones, and of dispensing from defining the etiology and the pathogenesis. As a matter of fact, this term should be reserved for atlantoaxial subluxations occurring without any apparent cause.

A historical review of atlantoaxial subluxation in chronic inflammatory rheumatism should also mention, besides rheumatoid arthritis, the other diseases.

In 1933, F.A.R. Stammers and P. Frazer [333] reported the case of a 30-year-old male with advanced ankylosing spondylarthritis complicated by pyramidal tract involvement and sensory disturbances. Treatment by extension and immobilization with a hard collar brought about regression of the troubles. C.W. Rand [285] reported in 1944 another case of ankylosing spondylarthritis showing a Brown-Séquard syndrome associated with atlantoaxial dislocation. Involvement of the cervical spine is a frequent finding in juvenile polyarthritis (34% of the cases). In 1957 S. Werne [396] published seven cases among which four, and perhaps even five, occurred in children with chronic polyarthritis. In 1962 W. Martel et al. [229] observed nine indisputable atlantoaxial subluxations among 17 children with cervical involvement. Up to now, only a few isolated cases have been reported in psoriatic arthropathy (W. Martel and J.W. Page, 1960 [230]; J. Sharp and D.W. Purser, 1961 [324]; V.J. Giuliano and T.J. Scully, 1972 [141]; M. Serre et al., 1963 [316]). Finally, to the author's knowledge, there exists no case report of craniovertebral region involvement in other inflammatory rheumatisms. Indeed, F.A.R. Stammers and P. Frazer's unique case [333] concerning such a lesion in a patient with ulcerous colitis, should be set apart.

Today, Davis and Markley's case is considered the first certain atlantoaxial subluxation encountered in rheumatoid arthritis. As a matter of fact, this report includes other data which have been partly disregarded up to recent years. In the introduction the authors state "... there was compression of the medulla oblongata by the odontoid process. The herniation of this process was secondary to destructive osseous changes of rheumatoid arthritis ..." Unfortunately, it had not been possible to perform X-rays. The post-mortem report does not mention the presence of anteroposterior atlantoaxial subluxation, but rather the upward subluxation with destruction of the atlas, the axis, and the occipital bone.

In 1952 Coste et al. [78] reported a case of anterior subluxation of the atlas on the axis in rheumatoid arthritis in a 35-year-old female. In 1955 G. Vignon and R. Patet [373] also reported a case occurring in rheumatoid arthritis. Later on, more cases were reported (S. de Sèze et al., 1957 [319]; G. Storey, 1958 [339]; Z. Kopera and A. Barwick-Schramm, 1960 [197]; F. Coste et al., 1960 [79]; W.B. Seanan and J. Wells, 1961 [313]). Finally, more general studies demonstrated the frequency of cervical spine involvement, and especially of the craniovertebral angle in rheumatoid arthritis. Thus, in 1958, J. Ball [19] found three subluxations among 18 postmortem examinations in rheumatoid arthritis. W. Martel and J.W. Page [230] carried out in 1960 a radioclinical study on about 24 cases. The prominent report of J. Sharp and D.W. Purser [324] was published the next year and concerned 48 cases of atlantoaxial subluxation among which 26 were associated with rheumatoid arthritis and 22 with ankylosing spondylarthritis.

At about the same time, surgical studies were published about craniovertebral arthrodesis and its indications in some atlantoaxial subluxations: T. Hauge [167], H.S. Dunbar and B.S. Rays [112], M. Lourie and W.A. Stewart [217], L. Rogers [293], J. Sharp and D.W. Purser [324], J. Dubousset et al. [111]. M. Cibert et al. [70] reported seven cases with posterior cervical graft.

The tomographic technique now allows one to visualize changes in different bone parts and to describe erosions, new bone formation, and also the different types of subluxations, namely, superior or upward luxation of the atlas, backward displacement of the atlas on the axis, backward displacement of the occipital bone on the atlas. If, at the beginning, only a few cases were known, larger recorded series are now available. Finally, in 1971, I.C. Isdale and P.W. Conlon [182] carried out studies in a larger number of cases and paid particular regard to the evolution of the anatomic changes in the craniovertebral joints, whereas J.C. Stevens et al. [336] paid special attention to neurological complications. These latter studies have opened up a new field for the treatment of this disease.

Part 2 Anatomy and Physiology of the Craniovertebral Region

Chapter 1 Osteology and Arthrology

Three bones constitute the craniovertebral region:

1. The occipital bone with its condyles
2. The atlas (anterior and posterior arches and lateral masses)
3. The axis (odontoid process, body of the axis, and the transverse process)

These three "bones of the hinge" constitute together six joints which control the very complex mobility of the craniovertebral region. We shall describe the following connections: the occipitoatlantal, occipitoaxial, and the connection between the two first vertebrae.

In this field we shall also report postmortem findings in arthrography.

I. Joint Between Occipital Bone and Atlas

By means of its lateral masses, the atlas articulates with the condyles of the occipital bone and forms the occipitoatlantal joint properly speaking. Moreover, the arches of both bones are distantly connected by the anterior and posterior occipitoatlantal ligaments.

A. Atlanto-Occipital Joint(s)

Articular Surfaces. These are, on the one hand, the condyles of the occipital bone and on the other the glenoid grooves of the atlas. The articular surfaces are covered with a thin layer of cartilage, which is thicker on the atlas than on the occipital bone.

Means of Union. A quite loose fibrous capsule, attached to the articular margins, connects them. Posteriorly and laterally, it is strengthened by the lateral occipitoatlantal ligaments. Frontally the capsule is continuous with the anterior occipitoatlantal ligament and posteriorly with the posterior occipitoatlantal ligament.

Synovial Membrane. Each atlanto-occipital condylarthrosis possesses a synovial membrane which is loose and has an inward extension that covers the upper margin of the transverse ligament near its attachment and fills the groove located on the internal aspect of the lateral masses, behind the attachment tubercle of this ligament.

B. Atlanto-Occipital Ligaments

Anterior and posterior atlanto-occipital ligaments connect distantly the anterior and posterior arches of the atlas with the occipital bone.

1. Anterior Atlanto-Occipital Ligament. It is laterally very thin and strengthened in the median plane by a fibrous membrane. During extension of the head, the median part stretches before the lateral fibers. Its development accounts for the part it plays in the obviation of these movements. The median fibers are covered by a fibrous cord which constitutes the origin of the anterior longitudinal ligament of the spine.

2. Posterior Atlanto-Occipital Ligament. It is thin and fibrous and connects the posterior margin of the foramen magnum with the upper edge of the posterior arch of the atlas. This ligament stretches only in exaggerated flexion of the head.

II. Connection Between Occipital Bone and Axis

The occipital bone and the axis have no articular contact but they are distantly connected by very strong ligaments. These are situated within the vertebral canal where they line the anterior wall and may be divided into two groups; one extending from the occipital bone to the body of the axis and forming the occipitoaxoid ligament, and the other joining the occipital bone to the odontoid process and termed the occipitodental ligaments.

A. Median Occipitoaxoid Ligament (Membrana Tectoria)

The membrana tectoria is a broad fibrous band which covers the dens and its ligaments. It has an important thickening in its median part and becomes progressively thinner toward the external borders. The numerous fibers of the middle layer blend on one hand with the cranial dura mater and on the other hand extend into the basilar groove above the margins of the foramen magnum. The fibers of the external band extend to the upper rim of the anterior margin of the foramen magnum and reach the occipital condyles. Caudally, this membrane becomes less broad and is continuous with the posterior longitudinal ligament of the spine. The latter appears to cover equally the intraspinal aspect of all cervical vertebrae. Its upper edge is attached to the occipital bone. In fact, the deep lamella is attached to the lower third of the intraspinal aspect of the body of the axis. The median occipitoaxial ligament controls the movements of dorsi and ventriflexion, the range of which is small in the occipitoatlantal joint since these movements not only occur at this level but in all articulations of the cervical spine. The membrana tectoria is located between the meninges and the spinal cord on the one hand and the occipitoatlantoaxoid ligamentous apparatus on the other and appears to be at once protective and restrictive. Numerous authors describe the lateral occipitoaxoid ligaments as part of the membrana tectoria. Hecker [169], however, describes them as individual structures, which seems logical. Indeed, the membrana tectoria limits the ventri and dorsiflexion movements, whereas the lateral occipitoaxoid ligaments control the rotation movements. They extend between the occipital condyles and the external part of the body of the axis on its spinal aspect.

B. Occipitodental Ligaments

The deep layer of the ligamentous apparatus connecting the odontoid process with the occipital bone consists of three ligaments, i.e., the lateral occipitodental ligaments or alar ligaments, and the median apical-odontoid ligament.

1. Lateral Occipitodental Ligaments (Alar Ligaments)

Their fibers extend from the lateral parts of the foramen magnum to the postero-lateral upper part of the dens. Sometimes the fibers form a transverse ligamentous band, curvilinear and upwardly concave and joining both occipital condyles.

These ligaments check the rotation of the head and thus take part in stabilization of the head on the spine. Since the occipital bone is connected with the odontoid process by these very strong ligaments, the atlas is maintained between the occipital bone and the axis. The fixation of the head on the axis by the alar ligaments hinders neither the rotation nor the flexion movements. However, in the case of extreme or forced rotation, the occipital condyles move further away from the odontoid process and stretch the alar ligaments to the utmost. As to the function of the transverse band, if any, it prevents dorsiflexion.

2. Median Apical-Odontoid Ligament (Ligamentum Apicis Dentis)

The apical ligament of the dens extends from the tip of the process to the middle of the anterior edge of the foramen magnum. It is inconstant and may be very poorly developed, simply strengthening cranially and dorsally the synovial capsule of the anterior atlanto-odontoid joint.

III. Connection Between Atlas and Axis

The two first vertebrae are connected medially (Fig. 1) and laterally. In the median part, the second cervical vertebra by means of its odontoid process projects into an osteofibrous ring formed by the anterior arch of the atlas and by a ligament arching from one lateral mass of the atlas to the other: the transverse ligament. The dens articulates ventrally with the osseous part and dorsally with the fibrous part of the ring. We shall study successively: (1) the joint between the anterior arch of the atlas and the anterior aspect of the odontoid process or *anterior atlantodental joint*; and (2) the *transverse ligament* and its articulation with the posterior aspect or *syndesmo-odontoid articulation.*

Laterally, the atlas is in contact with the superior articular processes by means of the inferior articular surfaces of its lateral masses. thus forming the atlantoaxoid articulation.

Moreover, the two vertebrae are connected by distant ligaments, i.e. the anterior and posterior atlantoaxial ligaments.

A. Anterior Atlantodental Joint

The joint between the anterior arch of the atlas and the anterior facet of the dens is a trochoid articulation.

Articular Surfaces. The posterior aspect of the anterior arch of the atlas bears on its median part an oval-shaped, slightly concave articular facet with the long axis passing transversely.

The anterior aspect of the dens bears an articular facet which is larger. This facet is oval-shaped, slightly convex; its long axis is vertical.

Both facets are covered with cartilage which is thicker on the dens than on the atlas.

Means of Union. A loose capsule joins the two surfaces. It is attached all around the margins of the articular facets, except for the superior pole of the odontoid facet,

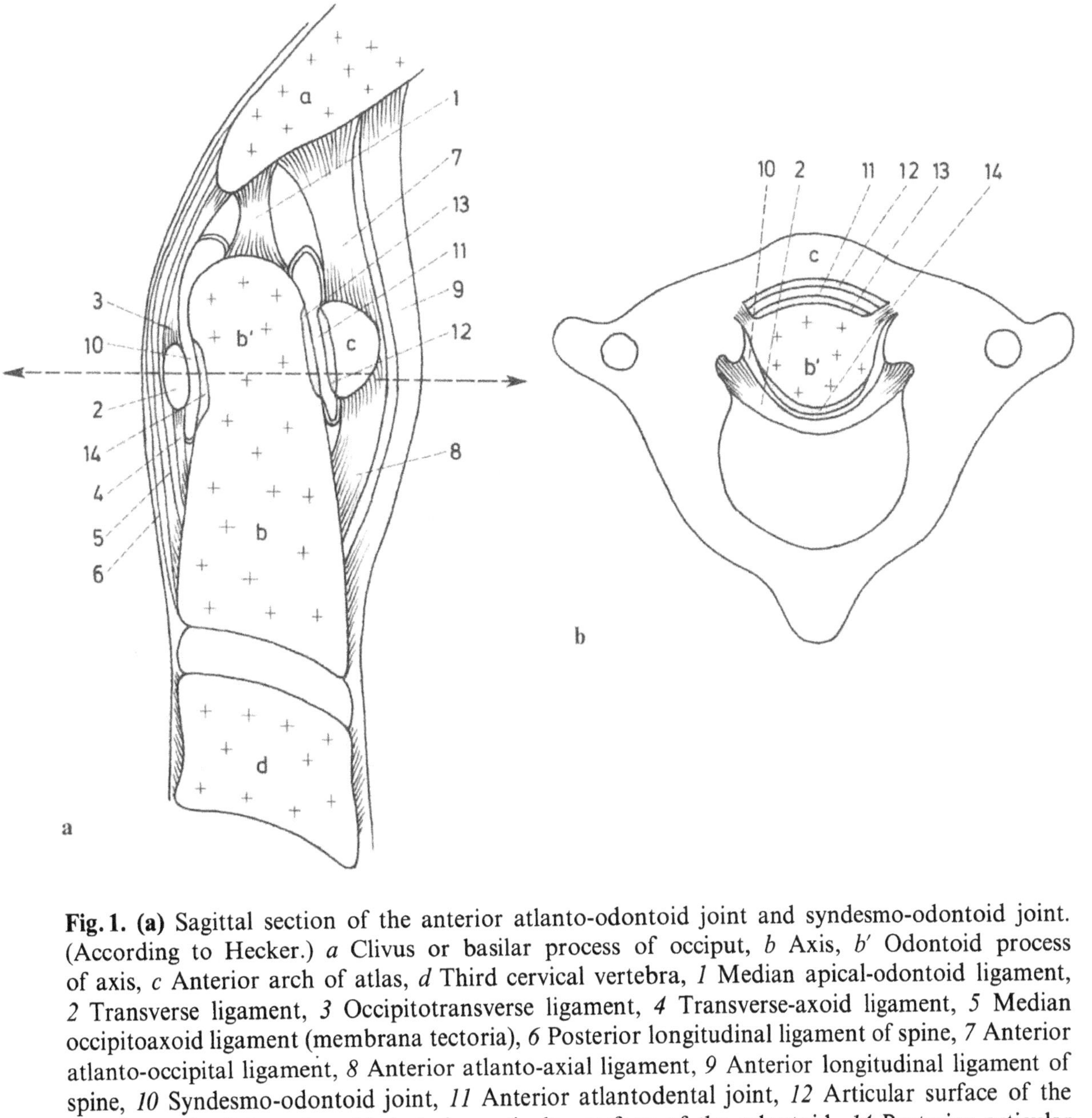

Fig. 1. (a) Sagittal section of the anterior atlanto-odontoid joint and syndesmo-odontoid joint. (According to Hecker.) *a* Clivus or basilar process of occiput, *b* Axis, *b′* Odontoid process of axis, *c* Anterior arch of atlas, *d* Third cervical vertebra, *1* Median apical-odontoid ligament, *2* Transverse ligament, *3* Occipitotransverse ligament, *4* Transverse-axoid ligament, *5* Median occipitoaxoid ligament (membrana tectoria), *6* Posterior longitudinal ligament of spine, *7* Anterior atlanto-occipital ligament, *8* Anterior atlanto-axial ligament, *9* Anterior longitudinal ligament of spine, *10* Syndesmo-odontoid joint, *11* Anterior atlantodental joint, *12* Articular surface of the anterior arch of the atlas, *13* Anterior articular surface of the odontoid, *14* Posterior articular surface of the odontoid. **(b)** Horizontal section of atlantodental and syndesmo-odontoid articulations

where it is continuous with the median apical odontoid ligament.

Synovial Membrane. It stretches slightly—about 2 mm—above and below the articular surfaces forming two small culs-de-sac, one superiorly and the other inferiorly. At this level, it is separated from the syndesmo-odontoid synovial membrane only by the thickness of the capsule.

B. Syndesmo-Odontoid Joint

It possesses the peculiarity of consisting of an anterior bony surface; the odontoid process: and a posterior ligamentous surface: the transverse ligament.

Transverse Ligament (Fig. 2). This ligament forms the fibrous part of the ring which retains the dens in contact with the anterior

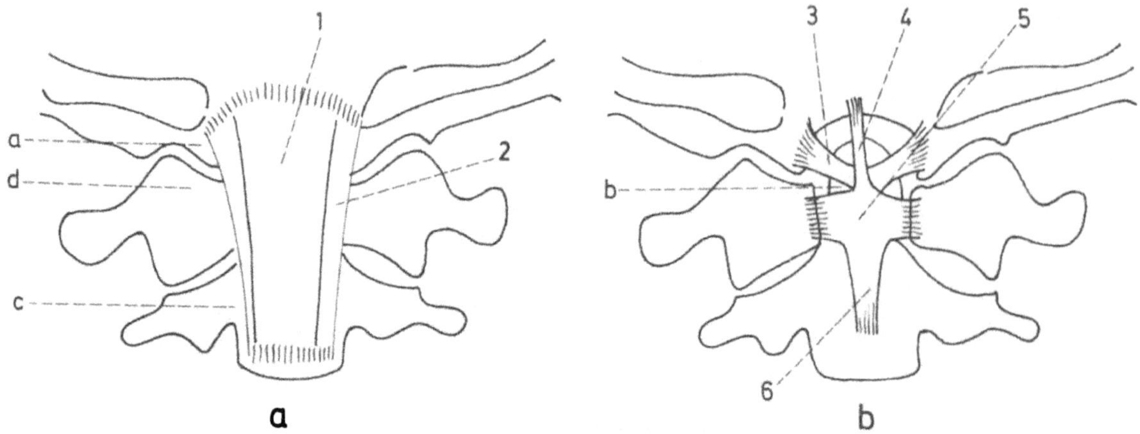

Fig. 2a and b. Intraspinal ligaments. **(a)** Superficial layer. **(b)** Middle layer. *a* Occipital condyle, *b* Odontoid process, *c* Body of axis, *d* Lateral mass of atlas, *1* Membrana tectoria, *2* Lateral occipitoaxoid ligament, *3* Alar ligament, *4* Occipitotransverse ligament, *5* Transverse ligament, *6* Transverse-axoid ligament

arch. It arches from one lateral mass of the atlas to the other, and is attached to the tubercle of the transverse ligament. It is cylindrical at the level of its attachments and becomes flat toward the midline where it is a band with concave anterior aspect, convex posterior aspect and two margins—superior and inferior.

The anterior aspect is transversely concave and contacts by its median part, the posterior articular facet of the odontoid process. The latter surface is lined with cartilage. The corresponding part of the transverse ligament is lined with a 6–8-mm-thick chondroid layer. The posterior aspect is continuous with the deep fibers of the occipitoaxoid ligament, except where they are kept apart by a synovial cavity or bursa, which is constant but of variable size.

A small flat band arises upward and forms the *occipitotransverse ligament.*

Another band extends downward and is attached to the posterior aspect of the body of the axis; it is the *transversary-axoid ligament.*

Hence, these two ligaments form a cross with the transverse ligament, which accounts for the term "cruciform ligament." The main function of this ligament is to form, together with the anterior arch of the atlas, the osteofibrous ring retaining the dens. The ascending band checks the ventriflexion movements and increase the stability of the transverse part. The descending band prevents the upward gliding of the transverse ligament and limits the ventriflexion movements of the skull on the upper cervical vertebrae. As to the Gruber ligament, it contributes to retaining the odontoid process in the atlantal ring and thus constitutes a complementary attachment of the transverse ligament.

Synovial Membrane. The posterior synovial membrane is larger than the anterior in the transverse as well as in the vertical axis. Inferiorly to the transverse ligament, it forms a small diverticulum, 3–4 mm high. Superiorly, it covers the posterior aspect of the dens up to the tip. Usually it terminates at the level of the attachment of the apical ligament of the dens, which is inconstant, and strengthens upward and posteriorly the synovial cavity of the anterior atlantodental joint. The synovial membrane may extend on both sides to the anterior arch of the atlas and communicate inconstantly with the antero-internal part of the corresponding atlantoaxial joint or with the anterior atlantodental joint. Some authors, and especially Werne [396], report the presence of a serous bursa between the odontoid process and the clivus (bursa apicis dentis). Fick [125] describes a case which he observed in 1884, in which the bursa mucosa apicis dentis was separated by a septum from the upper cul-de-sac of the syndesmo-odontoid synovia.

C. Atlantoaxial Joint(s)

This joint is a diarthrosis, type arthrodia. In a sense, it is a double joint as it consists of two separate and symmetrical articulations.

Articular Surfaces. They are formed by the inferior articular facets of the lateral mass of the atlas and by the superior articular processes of the axis. The articular surfaces are lined with cartilage, which is thicker toward the center and may measure 1.5 cm.

Means of Union. A loose fibrous capsule maintains the contact between those two surfaces. Medially, this capsule is strengthened by a fibrous band belonging to the occipitoaxoid ligament, known as *Arnold's ligament or lateral atlantoaxoid ligament.*

Synovial Membrane. A synovial membrane lines the internal aspect of the capsule. Sometimes it is continuous with the synovial membrane of the syndesmo-odontoid joint and another prolongation may run in front of the neck of the odontoid process to the atlanto-odontoid capsule.

D. Atlantoaxial Ligaments

The anterior arch of the atlas is connected with the anterior aspect of the body of the axis by a very thin fibrous lamina, medially strengthened, the *anterior atlantoaxial ligament.*

The posterior atlantoaxial ligament is a thin fibrous lamina joining the inferior edge of the posterior arch of the atlas to the base of the spinous processes of the axis.

Table 1. Functions of the intraspinal ligaments

Name	Function
Median occipitoaxial ligament	Checks flexion-extension in the occipitoatlantal joints
Lateral occipitoaxial ligaments	Check rotation of the head. Stabilize the head on the spine by preventing lateroflexion movements
Lateral occipitodental ligaments	Check rotation of the head. Stabilize the head on the spine. Prevent backward subluxation of the odontoid
Median apical-odontoid ligament	Suspension of the odontoid
Transverse ligament	Maintains the odontoid in contact with the anterior arch of the atlas
Occipitotransverse ligament Transverse-axoid ligament	Stabilize the transverse ligament
Lateral atlantoaxoid ligaments	Checks the rotation movements of the head. Reinforce the capsules of the atlantoaxial joints

Chapter 2 Normal Radiographic Anatomy

I. Normal Radiographic Anatomy of the Joint Spaces

It is far more difficult to visualize, radiologically, joint space lesions than bone lesions. Apart from the atlanto-odontoid joint which may be sometimes perfectly visualized on lateral projections, joints are best analyzed on frontal or lateral tomograms. The standardized tomographic methods work perfectly under normal anatomic conditions. This is, however, not the case with pathological conditions, as we shall see.

A. Atlanto-Occipital Joints

The correct projection for visualizing this particularly narrow space is frontal tomography. Indeed, it is almost impossible to obtain a good picture with plain X-rays. Apart from the anterior third, the articular interspace is only about 1 mm wide. Correct paramedian sagittal tomography also provides satisfying information but, on account of the articular orientation, i.e. from medially outward and from the front backward, several sections are necessary to visualize the entire articulation. The normal features of the articulations and the artifacts have been perfectly studied by von Torklus and Gehle [361], and by Wackenheim [380]. We would like to draw attention to the rather frequent occurrence of variants (platycondylia, brachycondylia, occipitalization, and vertebralization), and especially to the division into two parts of the glenoid articular surface of the atlas as well as of the condyle, as depicted in Rauber-Kopsch's anatomy. In this case, the anterior part is larger than the posterior; such a picture should not be taken for a subchondral bone lesion, but should be known as a normal variant (bilobed condyles).

B. Anterior Atlanto-Odontoid Joint

Only this part of the atlanto-odontoid joint is visible. Indeed, the syndesmo-odontoid joint, situated behind the odontoid process, is not visible since one of its constituants, the transverse ligament, is radiotransparent. Only indirect signs allow the recognition of arthritis at this level.

The configuration of this joint is variable. Usually, it has a slight anterior convexity. The normal range of width of this joint is rather great, widening being an excellent indirect sign of incompetence or damage to the transverse ligament. Measurement should be done on strictly median sagittal tomograms since the joint widens laterally.

In children, the space is larger than in adults, owing to the physiological hyperlaxity. However, according to some authors, this wider space would be due rather to a thicker cartilage. Only between the ages of 9 and 15 does the atlanto-odontal space acquire the adult width of 1–2 mm.

Narrowings of this space are difficult to evaluate, even on tomograms. The case report by Serre et al. [315] demonstrates this by a clear discrepancy between the radiological data consistent with the presence of a real interspace between the anterior arch of the atlas and the odontoid process on one hand, and the anatomical verification showing complete fusion of these parts and total absence of movement in the atlanto-odontoid joint on the other. It is very likely that the interspace had been replaced by less dense bone.

C. Lateral Atlantoaxial Joints

This articulation may be well visualized on plain a-p X-rays, and is usually not visible on lateral views. As concerns lateral tomograms, the shape of the articulation causes the space to appear wider posteriorly and anteriorly than in the middle. On frontal sections, however, it is wider in its middle part. One can only speak of a narrowing of the articular interspace, when it is visualized on several frontal and lateral projections. It should also be emphasized that the tomographic sections must be performed in a strictly symmetrical position of the head. Indeed, rotation of the head of more than 5° produces artifactitious changes in the interspace and may lead to misinterpretation, i.e., false narrowings.

II. Normal Radiographic Anatomy of the Bones

Let us recall here that conventional X-rays are usually not sufficient for a complete analysis and that tomograms are most of the time, if not always, necessary for a correct visualization of the bones in this region.

A. Occiput

1. Basilar process
2. Inferior occipital squama, which belongs to the craniovertebral angle region
3. Foramen magnum
4. Condylar area
5. Paracondylar area
6. Retrocondylar area
7. Cranial sutures

B. Atlas

1. Anterior arch of the atlas
2. Lateral masses and transverse process
3. Posterior arch of the atlas
4. Vertebral canal of the atlas

C. Axis

1. Body of the axis
2. Odontoid process
3. Pedicles
4. Articular processes
5. Laminae
6. Spinous process
7. Transverse processes
8. Bony canal

We shall not provide here a detailed study of all these bones but refer the reader to Wackenheim's monograph [380].

III. Angles, Lines and Bony Landmarks

I shall dispense with a description of all the geometrical landmarks in the cervico-occipital region. Normal values and their variations have been reported on in detail by Wackenheim [380]. There are numerous angles, lines, and landmarks quoted in this book, and we shall merely point out those used in current practice and those which are most often reported.

A. Lateral Projection

1. Basilar line (Thiebaut, Wackenheim and Vrousos)
2. Nasion–external protuberance line (Prouzet and James)
3. Height of posterior cranial fossa (Klaus)
4. Palato-occipital line (Chamberlain)
5. Palato-suboccipital line (McGregor)
6. Foramen magnum line (McRae)
7. Atlanto-palatine angle (Bull)
8. Atlanto-temporo-maxillary index (Fischgold, Lièvre and Simon)
9. Basio-odontoid index (Wholey, Bruwer and Baker)

B. Frontal Projection

1. Bimastoid line (Fischgold and Metzger)
2. Bidigastric line (Fischgold and Metzger)
3. Condylar angle (Schmidt and Fischer)
4. Intervestibular line (Wackenheim)

Chapter 3 Positive Arthrography of the Craniocervical Joints

Only a thorough knowledge of anatomy will allow correct analysis of bone anomalies in the craniocervical joints in rheumatoid arthritis. The site of these lesions depends on the features of the synovial cavity. They are mostly seen at the level of the insertions or of the synovial folds. This study is aimed at the radiological visualization of shape and volume of the articular cavities and of the communications between them.

I. Material and Method

The arthrograms were performed on unprepared autopsy specimens taken from subjects without chronic inflammatory rheumatism. The removal is done by the endocranial approach. A quadrangular section is removed at the level of the sella turcica, posteriorly to the foramen magnum and laterally with regard to perpendicular planes passing through the foramen ovale and the posterior condylar foramen. Then, by the anterior cervical approach, the cervical block is released from its muscular insertions and the cervical spine is severed below the third cervical vertebra. The cervical segment is carrefully dissected and the articular capsules are located.

The same technique is used with postmortem specimens for a study of the pathological changes in the craniocervical joints in chronic inflammatory rheumatisms. After numerous tests, the retained contrast medium is a mixture of one part Horsley's hemostatic wax and one part monoiodostearate ethyl ester, 32% iodine content wt/vol. This mixture is heated to color change and immediately injected, through a previously implanted needle, into the articulation.

All articulations of the craniocervical hinge, except for the syndesmo-odontoid joint, were thus injected.

II. Results

What conclusions can be drawn from the study of 18 specimens taken from adult subjects of both sexes and different ages?

A. Atlanto-Occipital Joints
(Fig. 3a, b)

Gray and Goss [148] point out the quite frequent existence of a communication between this joint and the atlanto-odontoid joint. Our experience does not allow us to agree. According to Testut and Latarjet [353] and to Poirier et al. [275] each occipitoatlantal condylarthrosis possesses, especially inwardly, a very loose synovial membrane where it continues more or less far over the odontoid ligaments and onto the

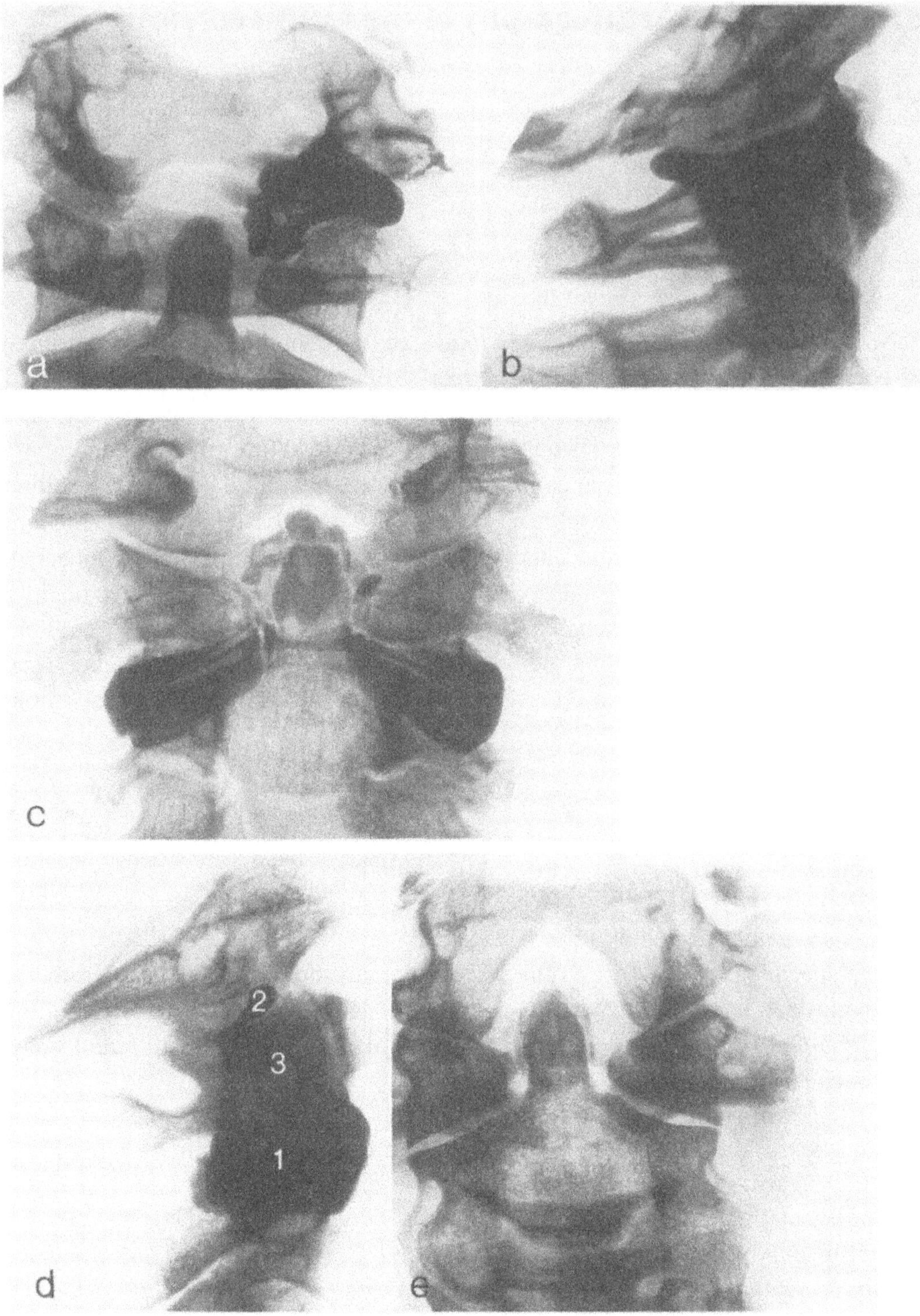

Fig. 3a–e. Arthrograms of the cranio-cervical joints. **(a)** Left atlanto-occipital joint in frontal view, **(b)** Atlanto-occipital joint in lateral view, **(c)** Injection in the left atlantoaxoid articulation. At the same time the right atlantoaxoid joint, the atlantodental and the syndesmodental joints are opacified, **(d)** Communication between the atlantoaxoid and the syndesmodental joints, **(e)** Paradental opacities due to opacification of the anterior atlantodental joint

superior margin of the transverse ligament, filling the groove situated at the internal aspect of the lateral masses, behind the insertion tubercle of this ligament. On our specimens we did not find the above-mentioned continuations. Contrariwise, we saw a very loose synovial membrane frontally, posteriorly, and, though less marked, outwardly. This laxity allows the flexion-extension movements.

B. Atlantoaxoid Joints

(Fig. 3c, d, e)

A very loose synovial membrane, especially frontally, favours the gliding of the articular surfaces. Testut describes two synovial folds, an anterior and a posterior one, progressing like two wedges into the dihedric angles formed by the superimposed articular facets of the atlas and of the axis. Because of the opaque contrast used, we could not provide evidence of such intraarticular synovial folds, even with tomograms.

The atlantoaxoid synovial membrane communicates quite frequently, by means of prolongations, with one or the other of the two synovial membranes of the atlantodental joint. The first prolongation runs toward the anterior aspect of the odontoid neck and sometimes communicates with the atlantodental articulation. The second runs toward the posterior aspect of the odontoid neck and often communicates with the transversodental synovial membrane. Thus, injection into the left atlantoaxoid articulation caused opacification of the right atlantoaxoid articulation, because both, the atlantodental and the syndesmodental articulations, are opacified at the same time. Sometimes only the atlantodental articulation communicates with the atlantoaxoid articulation and this seems to be the most frequent eventuality.

C. Atlantodental Joints

According to some, there is only one articulation. But others, including ourselves, are of the opinion that there are two distinct articulations, namely:

1. Anterior Atlanto-Dental Joint. The injection of this joint is difficult owing to the very narrow articular interspace. However, by injecting this joint we could opacify the syndesmodental joint. The contrast medium passes around the tip of the odontoid and descends along its posterior aspect. A bursa apicis dentis has been described between the clivus and the tip of the odontoid. There is perhaps such a bursa but we could never opacify it by means of intra-articular injections.

The synovial membrane extends above and below the articular surfaces but especially laterally where it largely covers the odontoid process and is seen on a-p X-rays as paradental opacities. According to Gaupp, quoted by Poirier et al. [275], in a great number of mammals the atlantodental synovial membrane communicates widely with the two atlantoaxial and atlanto-occipital synovial membranes. Thus, the five joints have the same cavity. As the mobility of the head on the cervical spine increases, the different synovial membranes become individualized. It is the pentacelom type.

2. Syndesmo-Odontoid Joint. This joint has a very reduced size. According to Kapandji [191] it is not a true articular cavity but rather a cellulo-adipose space which makes gliding possible. According to Poirier et al., the syndesmodental synovial membrane forms a large cavity without a proper articular capsule. As a matter of fact, our dissections and arthrographies showed the presence of a true articular cavity. This articulation is rather well developed above and below the transverse ligament, whereas at the very level of the ligament it is a virtual slit. In the neutral position and in flexion no contrast medium is to be seen between the odontoid and the transverse ligament, which is in close contact with the posterior articular facet. Laterally, this articulation continues onto the lateral aspect of the odontoid process and comes close to the atlantodental capsule. As to its eventual communication with the atlantoaxoid articulation, we mentioned this possibility above.

Chapter 4 Mechanics of the Joints

The cervical spine consists of two anatomically and functionally distinct parts:

The upper cervical spine comprises the first and second cervical vertebrae. These osseous parts are connected to each other and to the skull by an articular complex having three axes and three degrees of freedom.

The lower cervical spine stretches from the inferior aspect of the axis to the first thoracic vertebra. The articulations of the lower cervical spine allow two types of movements: flexion-extension and combined lateroflexion-rotation.

Functionally, the two segments are complementary in performing pure movements of rotation, lateroflexion, ante- and retroflexion, and forward and backward sliding.

I. Flexion-Extension Movement in the Atlantoaxial and Atlanto-Odontoid Joints

During flexion-extension movement, the transverse ligament retains the anterior arch of the atlas in close contact with the odontoid process. Consequently, the inferior facet of the lateral masses of the atlas tilts and glides at the same time on the superior aspect of the axis. The presence of the transverse ligament, which forms the posterior part of the atlanto-odontoid joint, allows a certain smoothness in the function of this articulation. This ligament, embedded in the posterior groove of the odontoid process, may curve either upward during extension or downward during flexion like the drawstring of a bow.

II. Rotation in the Atlantoaxial and Atlanto-Odontoid Joints

The atlanto-odontoid joint is a trochoid or pivot joint, comprising two cylindrical surfaces encased one into the other. These are – the odontoid process, an almost cylindrical pivot which allows the joint to adapt to a second degree of freedom during flexion-extension movement; and the osteoligamentous ring, formed ventrally by the anterior arch of the atlas, laterally by the lateral masses and dorsally by the transverse ligament.

During a rotation movement, the ring moves around the dens. Simultaneously there occurs a displacement in both atlantoaxoid joints. However, the superior surfaces of the axis are postero-anteriorly convex. Thus, the displacement of the lateral masses is not linear in a horizontal plane but curvilinear with upper convexity.

III. Rotation in the Atlanto-Occipital Joints

When the occipital bone rotates on the atlas it participates in a general rotation movement of the atlas on the axis, which occurs around the vertical axis passing through the center of the odontoid process. However, this rotation produces stretching of the ligaments and especially of the lateral odonto-occipital ligament. Thus, rotation is accompanied by concomitant displacement toward the same side and by obliquity of the occipital bone to the right. Consequently, there is no pure rotation, but rotation associated with translation and lateroflexion. The real center of the rotation is displaced toward the center of the foramen magnum so that the real axis of the rotation movement corresponds to the anatomical axis of the medulla oblongata.

IV. Lateroflexion and Anteretroflexion in the Atlanto-Occipital Joints

The range of *lateroflexion* is very small and results in a gliding of the occipital condyles on the lateral masses of the atlas (whereas there is no displacement in the atlantoaxoid joint). During this movement one of the condyles draws nearer to the odontoid process without ever coming into contact, since the movement is restricted by the stretching of the capsule of the atlanto-occipital joint and especially by the lateral occipitodental ligament.

Ante- and retroflexion movements of the occipital bone on the atlas occur by a gliding movement of the occipital condyles on the lateral masses of the atlas. During flexion the occipital condyles move backward on the lateral masses of the atlas. Simultaneously, the squama of the occipital bone moves away from the posterior arch of the atlas and, since this movement is always accompanied by flexion in the atlantoaxoid joint, the posterior arch of the atlas also moves away from the posterior arch of the axis. Flexion is checked by the stretching of the capsules and of the posterior ligaments (occipitoatlantal membrane and posterior cervical ligament).

During *extension* the occipital condyles glide forward on the lateral masses of the atlas. Simultaneously, the squama of the occipital bone moves toward the posterior arch of the atlas and, since there also occurs an extension in the atlantoaxoid joint, the posterior arch of the atlas moves toward the posterior arch of the axis. Extension is restricted by the contact between these three osseous parts.

V. Sliding Movement

This movement consists of forward and backward displacement of the head with regard to the atlas-axis block. This movement is checked by the median apical odontoid ligament, the median occipitoaxoid ligament, and also by the posterior atlanto-occipital membrane. The displacement is only of a few degrees and no detailed anatomical study is available.

The *range of mobility* in different movements is depicted in the table below.

	Fick [125]	Poirier et al. [275]	Werne [396]
Atlanto-occipital joints			
Anteretroflexion	50°	50°	13°
Lateroflexion	30–40°	14–40°	8°
Sliding	Not mentioned		
Atlantoaxoid joints			
Anteretroflexion	Insignificant	11°	10°
Lateroflexion	0	4 mm	0
Rotation	60°	30–80°	47°

Chapter 5 Radiological Studies of the Mobility of the Joints

Functional examinations, thanks to modifications of the radiographic picture during movement, are indispensable in providing evidence of articular mobility. The best known of these dynamic tests is the flexion-extension movement, but lateroflexion, rotation, and sliding should also be taken into account.

I. Flexion-Extension

[208, 270, 287, 380, 381]

About 30% of the flexion-extension mobility of the cervical spine occur at the level of the cervico-occipital joints. We should like to emphasize that this examination demands very a strict technique. Indeed, at the end of the flexion movement, when the chin abuts against the sternum, some deflexion occurs at the level of the cervico-occipital joint. The maximal flexion of the upper cervical segment is only obtained by drawing the head as far back as possible and then tucking the chin in (Penning). This explains why some, for instance Wackenheim, recorded a diminution of the posterior occipitoatlantal interspace, between the occipital squama and the spinous process of the axis, during the spontaneous flexion movement.

The mobility in the cervico-occipital joints may be more accurately studied by means of different methods (Fig. 4);

Penning's method, type 1 and 2
Wackenheim's method
The author's method

A. Penning's Method [270]

In order to analyze the mechanism of movement of the cervical vertebrae, the corresponding two functional radiographs demonstrating the end-positions of each movement are combined to form the so-called movement diagram. Type 1 shows the upper vertebra in both end-positions of the movement, while the lower vertebra is in a fixed position (Fig. 4a). Type 2 shows the upper vertebra in a fixed position, while the lower vertebra shows both end-positions of the movement (Fig. 4b). The movement diagram of the CO/1 segment in the flexion-extension movement is constructed by superimposing the image of the atlas and tracing out the contours of the occiput. This is type 1. In type 2 the contours of the occiput are superimposed and those of the atlas traced out.

B. Wackenheim's Method [381]

Chamberlain's line is traced in the three positions; neutral, flexion, and extension. These three lines determine a triangular surface which characterizes the amplitude of the displacement of the head, the shape of

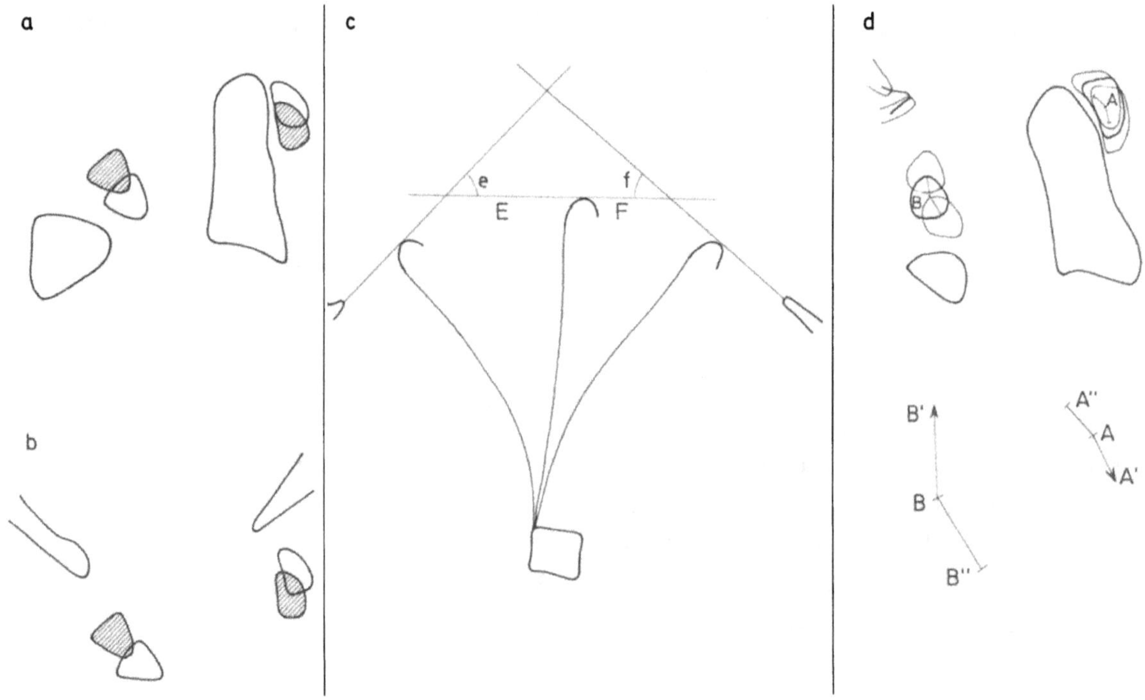

Fig. 4a–d. Methods of study of flexion-extension mobility in the cervicooccipital joints. **(a)** Penning's method, type I. **(b)** Penning's method, type II. **(c)** Wackenheim's method. **(d)** Author's method. Diagram of the mobility of the anterior and posterior arch of the atlas. Point *A* corresponds to the center of the anterior arch of the atlas, *A′* to displacement in flexion, *A″* to displacement in extension. Point *B* corresponds to the center of the posterior arch of the atlas

which indicates the degree of participation of the cervico-occipital joint in the flexion extension movement, when the movement is normal between C2 and C7. Under normal conditions, the triangle is approximately isosceles with a large surface (Fig. 4c).

C. Author's Method

The contours of the atlas and of the edges of the foramen magnum are traced with regard to the axis considered to be fixed. We determine the center of the anterior arch of the atlas (A) and the center of the posterior arch of the atlas (B). The displacement of these points (A – A′ – A″ and B – B′ – B″) determine vectors. Vector A A′ A″ normally materializes a movement of vertical component with slight gaping of the atlantodental interspace. Vector B B′ B″ shows the progressive gap between the spinous processes of C1 and C2 and the occipital squama (Fig. 4d).

Penning's method allows tracing of the movement diagram, i.e., the relationships between the vertebrae during the different phases of the movement, the amplitude of this movement, and its axis. Wackenheim's method is quicker and more useful as a daily routine. It provides data only about the mobility in the cervico-occipital joint considered as one block. The author's method, to be sure, takes more time but seems well adapted to the study of the mobility of the atlas and thus, to the diagnosis of the main lesions in chronic inflammatory rheumatisms, atlanto-odontoid subluxation. It may thus be considered as a method specific for rheumatology of the cervico-occipital joint.

II. Forward and Backward Sliding [382]

This examination provides evidence about the tension placed upon the occipitodental ligament and the tectorial membrane during forward and backward sliding movements. It would thus be useful to show subluxations and especially upward subluxations of the odontoid process. However, these movements are rather complex, i.e., forward sliding is combined with extension and backward sliding with flexion. We have no real experience with these movements in rheumatics.

III. Rotation [380]

Rotation of the upper cervical segment occurs normally only at the atlantoaxial joint and not at all, or at least very little, at the atlanto-occipital joints. Radiological analysis of the rotation of the atlas requires a perfectly symmetrical position of the axis. Over a rotation of 30° in the atlantoaxial joints, the axis itself starts to rotate jointly with the rest of the spine.

The signs of rotation of the atlas are the following:

1. The transverse processes of the atlas are well defined on one side and blurred on the other.
2. The lateral mass of the atlas is withdrawn with regard to the axis on the side that moves backward.
3. The atlantodental space is narrowed on the side that moves backward.
4. The size of the lateral mass of the atlas is diminished on the side that turns backward, owing to the optical projection of the more sagittally oriented lateral mass in the rotated position.

The analysis of the rotation image is useful for the correct interpretation of lateroflexion.

IV. Lateroflexion [380]

It is very important to obtain a pure lateroflexion movement in order to be able to give a correct interpretation of the X-ray. Lateroflexion must be very discreet, about 5 to 7°; beyond this, amplitude rotation would occur. To make sure that there is no rotation, a frontal tomogram is performed, which must visualize both vestibules on the same section.

The signs of lateroflexion are the following:

1. The joint between the occipital condyle and the lateral mass of the atlas is narrowed on the tilted side and enlarged on the opposite side.
2. The lateral margin of the atlas overlaps the margin of the axis on the tilted side.
3. The atlanto-odontoid interspace is asymmetrical, narrowed on the side of lateroflexion and enlarged on the other side.

These dynamic examinations are not all used in current practice. Only the flexion-extension examination is usually carried out. This provides, moreover, the most important data for the diagnosis as well as for treatment.

Part 3 Pathological Anatomy

If anatomopathological lesions of the cervico-occipital joints in rheumatoid arthritis have been fairly well studied, only little is known in this area for the other chronic rheumatic diseases.

The first description of a lesion in the cervico-occipital joints in rheumatoid arthritis was that of Davis and Markley [89]. Their report stated: "On examination of the base of the skull from above, there was an obvious mass, about 1 cm in diameter, raised 0.5 cm above the surface of the occipital bone just in front of the foramen magnum. This mass clearly impinged on the inferior surface of the medulla, forming a definite depression there and compressing this structure significantly at a point just below the pons. Sagittal section of this bony region showed the mass to be the odontoid process which had herniated upwards through the foramen magnum. The anterior arch of the atlas and possibly a portion of the occipital bone immediately surrounding this process were soft, appearing to be replaced by both fibrous and necrotic tissue. The overlying dura was smooth. Microscopic sections of the region of the herniated odontoid process showed evidence of bone destruction and fragmentation as well as fibrosis and new bone formation. Several areas of fresh collagen necrosis typical of active rheumatoid disease were seen both here and in sections of other joints."

For our anatomopathological study we reviewed all publications including postmortem examinations of patients deceased from lesions in the cervico-occipital joints in rheumatoid arthritis. Besides the abovementioned case of Davis and Markley, we counted 14 other cases: Storey [339], Martel and Page, 1960 [230], Martel and Abell, 1963 [226], Serre et al., 1963 [315], Gleason and Urist, 1965 [142], Verjaal and Hardner, 1965 [368], Bland, 1967 [31], Webb et al., 1968 [390], and Cibert [69]. The publications of Eulderink and Meijers, 1971 [118], and Meijers et al., 1974 [246], who reported some anatomic findings without defining the number of cases with autopsy, should also be mentioned. Finally, papers such as those by Kao et al. [190] report anatomopathological findings recorded after surgery.

In rheumatoid arthritis the atlantoaxial, atlanto-odontoid and syndesmo-odontoid joints are involved by lesions which are quite comparable to those occurring in the peripheral articulations. They are primarily and mainly chronic inflammatory synovitis lesions. The capsuloligamentous, cartilaginous, and bone changes are secondary to the synovial lesions.

I. Articular Lesions

A. Rheumatoid Synovitis

Occurs and later predominates at the inner layer of the synovial membrane. It has no specific features but possesses some peculiarities. The first of them is a marked synovial proliferation. The internal wall of the synovial membrane is made of several cell layers instead of a single one. The underlying connective tissue becomes a highly vascularized granulation tissue. The villi of the synovial membrane are markedly hypertrophic. All along the articular interspace the proliferative synovial tissue forms a connective vascular process infiltrating the cartilage. This synovial pannus tends to extend to the center of the joint and thus to destroy the underlying cartilage. The second peculiarity in rheumatoid synovitis is the presence of numerous lymphocytic nodules within the inflammatory pannus. These are mainly made of lymphocytes but also of plasma cells and of histiocytes. These nodules are not pathognomonic.

Fibrinoid necrosis is frequent and may even develop into complete necrosis. Rheumatic vasculitis is not uncommon. Rheumatoid nodules are rather rare. A more or less abundant intra-articular exsudation may be seen in rheumatoid synovitis. The serous bursae, which are lined with synovial tissue, undergo the same changes as the articular synovia.

B. Capsular and Ligamentous Lesions

These have been studied mainly on the transverse ligament. The inflammatory granuloma of the transverse ligament provokes distention and, more rarely, rupture of this ligament. In the presence of a lax or ruptured ligament, the atlas vertebra slips forward; and in doing so, is aided by the convex configuration of the articular surfaces.

Werne [396] experimentally demonstrated on anatomic specimens that the forward luxation of the atlas is only possible when the transverse ligament is ruptured, and that, then, the anterior displacement is still checked by the alar ligament; the importance of the anterior atlanto-odontoid diastasis depends on the functional length of the alar ligament. On a series of 13 autopsies incompetence of the transverse ligament was only found in 3 cases (Martel and Abell [226]; Webb et al. [390]). Of these 3 patients, 2 died of upper cervical cord compression secondary to atlantoaxial subluxation. In the third patient, though the transverse ligament was ruptured, death was due to destruction of the lateral mass of the atlas with upward displacement of the odontoid process and bilateral vertebral artery occlusion.

However, other mechanisms, such as those responsible for Grisel's syndrome, could play a role. Berkheiser and Seidler [27] incriminate distention of the ligaments secondary to synovitis. As early as 1918 Jacobs [185] referred to "luxation-distention," a term that had also been used by Coste et al. [78] in their first case report. Greig [150] believes the main cause to be hyperemia. This thesis has been backed by Watson-Jones [388]: chronic inflammation produces hyperemia and thus decalcification and disinsertion of the transverse ligament. According to Kao et al. [190], one of the causes of failure to reduce the atlantoaxial subluxation is the presence of rheumatoid granulation tissue between the anterior arch of the atlas and the odontoid process.

C. Lesions of Cartilage and Bone

They are not present in the early stages. Contrary to the synovial lesions, which are reversible, destructive lesions of cartilage and bone are irreversible.

Articular cartilages undergo a series of regressive changes. Moreover, they may be invaded in their deeper parts by an ingrowth of inflammatory connective tissue which develops in the subchondral osseous spaces. Also, the cartilages are probably altered by the proteolytic enzymes produced by the leukocytes in the articular effusion. Finally, the cartilages are almost completely destroyed.

The bone undergoes osteoporosis. At some foci the granulation tissue forms lacunae corresponding to the pseudocystic areas visible on the X-rays. As has already been mentioned, it may also erode the subchondral bone lamina and invade the cartilage from underneath. This is the mechanism of bone destruction. Arthritis usually ends up with fibrous ankylosis. Bone ankylosis is rare. H. Serre et al. [315] report a case with fusion of the anterior arch of the atlas with the odontoid process in which the articular interspace had disappeared. Most often, however, there are erosions and bone destruction.

The odontoid process may be eroded by the adjacent involvement of the synovia, either anteriorly, between the anterior arch of the atlas and the odontoid process, or posteriorly, between the posterior aspect of the odontoid process and the anterior aspect of the transverse ligament.

Martel and Abell's anatomical study provides a good description of these erosions [226].

Boyle [45] points out the possibility of erosive involvement of the odontoid tip which he attributes to the occasional presence of a serous bursa at the tip of the dens. Erosion of the clivus would be due to the same cause.

Gleason and Urist [142] also insist on the possibility of complete separation between the base of the odontoid process and the axis.

The occipital bone, the lateral masses of the atlas, and the upper articular processes of the axis may be destroyed. We have already quoted the case reported by Webb et al. and the case of Davis and Markley. The third case, with postmortem examination, is that of Martel and Page [230]. Such findings are common in radiologic examination.

II. Lesions of the Meninges

Gutmann and Hable [159] report a case of pachymeningitis and review five other cases in the literature. Pachymeningitis would be due to fibrosis. Arachnoiditis is also said to be frequently seen. Hopkins [180] gave a good description of this lesion, but in the lower cervical spine, and laid stress on the fact that it can be, by itself, responsible for cord compression. One could extrapolate to the existence of such lesions at the level of the cervico-occipital joint. No case of cord compression by a rheumatoid nodule has been reported in the cervico-occipital region. But Friedman [137] describes a case of compression in the lumbosacral segment, in which "the intraspinal nodule was found compressing the fifth lumbar and the first sacral root on the right. Histological examination showed on frozen section compatibility with the diagnosis of dermoid tumor or rheumatoid nodule. The permanent sections resembled a rheumatoid nodule. There was a marked histocytic reaction in all areas sectioned. Fibrinoid necrosis was present, with areas of necrosis surrounded by palisades of histiocytes and fibroblasts. Many giant cells and multinucleated forms were seen."

III. Medullary Compression

These different involvements of the soft parts may cause reduction of the spinal canal. However, cord compression is prominently caused by osseous changes with anterior luxation of the atlas. It goes without saying that any narrowing of the medullary canal, either fixed or intermittent, such as congenital anomaly of the odontoid and especially the so-called odontoideum mobile (Wackenheim [380]) with its backward subluxation, contributes to increase the risk of cord compression. Very recently, Chaouat and Kanovitch [67] described a case of atlantoaxial subluxation in severe rheumatoid arthritis with decompensated and up to then well-tolerated Chiari malformation.

IV. Lesions of the Vertebral Artery

Atlantoaxial subluxation may involve the vertebral artery by causing its course to become even more sinuous. Crellin et al. [83], Whaley and Dick [399] and especially Webb et al. [390] emphasize this fact. The latter authors report the following microscopic data: "Both vertebral arteries were blocked by thrombi at their upper ends where they followed a tortuous course among the disorganized collapsed remnants of the atlas and the axis."

V. Lesions of the Nervous Structures

These consist mainly in ischemic lesions of the nerve tissue whatever the underlying mechanism. Postmortem examinations carried out in several cases showed the following changes:

On gross examination, the compressed tissues undergo necrosis, the meningeal envelopes appear congested, edematous with foci of hemorrhage.

Microscopically, there is congestion and edema and small foci of hemorrhage which are responsible for some dilaceration of the nervous tissue. Contrariwise, there are no signs in favor of inflammatory lesions properly speaking. The involvement of vessels is variable, whether or not it represents the main mechanism, and may go from normal features to complete thrombosis of one or both vertebral arteries. Areas of atheromas are common findings in aged individuals and it is generally admitted that they may, together with the above-mentioned changes, favor the occurrence of neurological complications.

Part 4 Clinical Examination

Chapter 1 Rheumatologic Examination

Involvements of the craniovertebral joints by rheumatoid arthritis are characterized by the absence of specific clinical data; and the symptomatology, if any, is not greatly suggestive in the majority of cases.

Total absence of cervical signs is not uncommon. Serre et al. [316] observed 4 patients out of 23 presenting with atlantoaxial subluxation, who had no clinical signs. For Sharp and Purser [324] it was 6 out of 26. The subluxations without clinical features make up about 15% of the cases. Arthritis of the occipitoatlantal and atlantoaxoid joints may develop without clinical evidence. Moreover, if there are clinical features, it is almost impossible to decide which of them are due to the first or to the second of these two conditions. It is also very difficult to tell what is secondary to craniocervical joint involvement or to lower cervical spine involvement. The most frequent functional sign is neck pain. More or less long-standing and more or less moderate neck pain may be sometimes characteristic of craniocervical joint involvement. Usually these pains develop progressively but they may also start briskly. They are of suboccipital location radiating to the occiput and even to the temporal and frontal area, to the back or toward the shoulders. Their intensity is variable: often moderate, sometimes acute, and sometimes increasing during the night. Neck pains are provoked or aggravated by jarring, as that of a car ride for instance.

In marked upward subluxations of the odontoid process, examination may reveal a *shortened neck,* analogous to that seen in basilar invagination.

A certain stiffness of the neck, whether associated with pain or not, is often recorded. Consequently, the limitation of active mobility concerns rotation especially. Clinical examination of mobility of the neck usually awakens the pain. Flexion-extension is rarely involved, though extension may be partly restricted. Measurements, expressed in centimeters, of the distance of the chin-suprasternal notch allows follow-up of the evolution. Functional radiographs (Penning) also provide precise measurements. The degree of limitation in lateroflexion is difficult to appreciate since this movement is already of very small amplitude normally. As we already pointed out, these signs are unfortunately non-specific and may be due as well to involvement of the craniovertebral joint as to involvement of the lower cervical spine.

As a matter of fact, suggestive abnormal attitude is extremely rare. According to some, for instance Arlet et al. [9], de Sèze et al. [322], and Sharp and Purser [324], there would exist a triple displacement of the head, at once pushed forward, flexed on the neck with the chin close to the sternum and not easily raised, and flattening of the normal lordosis of the neck. Sometimes there is a slight rotation and lateroflexion of the head due to asymmetrical gliding of the articular facets. Palpable protrusion of the spinous process of the axis and anterior bulging of the atlas perceptible on pharyngeal palpation are classical but rare signs. Serre et al. often recorded pain on palpation of atlas and axis.

Sometimes the patient reports crepitus during flexion of the head, which can also be heard by the examiner. Thus, in one of our patients with a reducible atlantoaxoid subluxation we took functional X-rays in different positions of the head – before and after the crepitus – and could demonstrate that the noise which is perceived corresponds to the gap between the anterior arch of the atlas and the odontoid process (Fig. 81). This condition may provoke a *feeling of instability of the head*, which is, according to Brattström and Granholm [48], an indication for surgery.

The Sharp and Purser test is useful in some severe and mobile subluxations when there is only mild pain and muscular contracture. It is carried out as follows: "The palm of one hand was placed on the patient's forehead and the thumb of the other on the tip of the spinous process of the axis. The patient was then asked to relax the neck in a semi-flexed position. By pressing backwards with the palm, a sliding motion of the head backwards in relation to the spine of the axis could be demonstrated. The movement was usually only appreciated by the observer, but in one patient was also clearly visible." In his series of 100 cases of rheumatoid arthritis Stevens et al. [336] recorded a positive Sharp and Purser test in one case without subluxation and in 16 out of 36, i.e. in 44% of the cases with subluxation; so that he believes the test to have diagnostic value when it is positive. We found this test to be positive in about 20% of our cases and we think that the coexistence of arthritis in the atlantocondylar and atlantoaxoid joints with subluxation accounts for its being found inconstantly.

In conclusion, it is not possible to individualize a rheumatologic clinical syndrome in the cervico-occipital region. Nor is it possible, from a clinical point of view, to distinguish different types of subluxation. We shall bear in mind that even the most ambiguous cervical signs may go along with subluxations and that this may also be seen on a cervical spine free of any rheumatoid process.

Chapter 2 Neurologic Manifestations

Neurologic disturbances in lesions of the craniovertebral joint are secondary to the different types of subluxations. It is the more or less paroxysmal upper cervical cord compression that has drawn attention to such lesions which were unknown up to the first case report of Davis and Markley in 1951 [89]. Only then, did several authors systematically search for more discrete neurologic signs.

The neurological examination of a patient with rheumatoid arthritis can present difficulties in the case of severe arthritis or in the multi-operated patient. These patients are usually hyperesthetic and clumsy. They have deformed or ankylosed articulations so that the search for objective signs and their interpretation becomes difficult, especially since there may also exist other neurological involvements, such as multineuritis, myopathies or iatrogenic neuropathies, syndromes of the carpal or tarsal canals, and lower cervical myelopathies (Hart [164, 165]).

Arnold's neuralgia is a frequent finding in atlantoaxial subluxation and in upward luxation of the odontoid. Pain may be experienced on one or on both sides. It is usually permanent but may be aggravated by the movements of the head or even by walking. Its intensity is variable, but painful paroxysms are caused by movements of the neck or by a strain. Sometimes pain may be relieved by bed rest or by wearing a collar. Painful radiations toward the retroocular region may occur, since there may be anastomosis between the branches of C2 and the frontal branch of the trigeminal nerve.

Finally, there may also be hypoesthesia of one or all modes of the superficial sensibility of the greater occipital nerve.

The neurological signs of *pyramidal tract involvement* are numerous and of polymorphic character according to extent and severity. They are paralysis predominantly distal; spread or polykinetic deep tendon reflexes; sometimes with knee or ankle clonus; uni- or bilateral Babinski and Hoffmann signs; variously affected tone and muscle strength, and, sometimes, spasmodic movements of one or several limbs – whether spontaneous or provoked by different stimuli. The criteria of an objective pyramidal tract involvement vary according to various authors except for some general consensus. Diminution in tone and muscle strength are almost never taken into account unless they are of brisk onset; contrariwise, signs of spinal cord irritation, though very difficult to elicit are considered significant, while, according to Mathews [233] the only valuable signs of pyramidal tract involvement are the Babinski and Hoffmann signs, the other signs not being reliable enough. Serre et al. [316] elicited hyperreflectivity in 8 of their 22 cases with subluxation and in 10 of 37 cases without subluxation, but he finally considered only 2 cases as having pyramidal tract involvement secondary to atlantoaxial subluxation. Stevens et al. [336] discussed the significance of modifications in deep tendon reflexes. According to them the diagnosis of myelopathy is based only on the modifications in deep tendon reflexes. For their study the neurological examination was cross-checked by three examiners and carried out before X-rays of the neck had been taken, so as to avoid premature judgment as to the presence of atlantoaxial subluxation; subsequent to which a five-point grading system was adopted. Only grade 4 reflexes were regarded as pathological and not unless they had been so graded independently by the three examiners. In their series of 100 patients with rheumatoid arthritis of whom 36 had atlantoaxial subluxation, Stevens et al. found 24 to have pyramidal tract involvement. However, pyramidal signs were also present in 16% of the patients without atlantoaxial subluxation. Stevens et al. in reviewing Garrod [140], reported "... distinct increase of one or more of the reflexes in 32 out of 50 patients in whom [he] specifically examined the supinator, triceps and knee jerks." He went on to say that "the most excessive jerks were not infrequently obtained in cases in which the joints were the seat of advanced changes" and he describes several instances in which "the exaggeration is very remarkable, one patient having ankle clonus." As concerns the 10 patients who were found to have pyramidal signs without subluxation, Stevens et al. report that in 3 cases the symptomatology was probably related to a lower cervical spine involvement whereas the 7 other patients were thought to have had inflammatory hypertrophy of the soft parts that could have been proved only by myelography.

Vertebrobasilar insufficiency may produce a quite polymorphic clinical picture consisting of transitory disturbances of equilibrium with or without vertigo and tinnitus, transitory diplopia by paralysis of the third, fourth, or sixth nerve, transitory ischemia of the occipital lobe, positive visual phenomena, and transitory bilateral cortical blindness or hemianopia. Definite cases of vertebral artery involvement have been reported, assessed either by angiography or by autopsy which had disclosed stenosis or occlusion (Cregan [82], Hamblen [162], Martel [225], Webb et al. [390]).

The disturbances of subjective sensation affect especially the extremities and mainly the upper limbs: paresthesiae, numbness, tingling, appreciation of hot and cold stimuli, electricity-like sensations. They are particularly characteristic of upper cervical spine involvement when they are produced by sudden movements of the head and accompanied by neck pain – similar to Lhermitte's sign. Disturbances in deep sensation are demonstrated by the vibration and the postural sensibility tests. They most often affect the upper limbs and are responsible for astereognosia. Disturbances in superficial sensation are inconstant and of late onset. When present, they may affect all modalities but mostly the tactile sense. Meijers et al. [246] found these signs to have a complementary value when they are associated with pyramidal signs.

Rana et al. [283], in a series of 41 patients with atlantoaxial subluxation of 3 mm or more, found 8 patients who showed unequivocal signs of sensory impairment over the face. "Trigeminal nerve impairment was invariably in the first division. This strongly suggests involvement of the descending tract of the nerve, which reaches as low as the second cervical segment and could thus be damaged by a displaced dens. The trigeminal nerve may also be affected by vascular disease of the pons, but other signs may be present to elucidate the site of the lesions".

Bulbar disturbances are usually of paroxysmal onset and may be fatal. Such cases have been reported by Davis and Markley [89], Martel and Abell [226], Coste et al. [80], and Cibert et al. [70]. It may be acute cardiac and respiratory insufficiency, but sometimes also paralysis and labioglossopharyngeal amyotrophy or disturbances in swallowing and phonation. Dysphagia may be due to lower cervical subluxations as has been reported for instance by Saffouri and Ward [302] in a case with hyperostosis and osteoarthritis. The differential diagnosis between a neurological syndrome of bulbar origin and a mere mechanical obstruction is based on X-rays of the esophagus, on laryngoscopy, and on esophagiscopy. Martel [225], Sweetnam [348], and Boyle [45] found bulbar disturbances to be the cause of some unexplained deaths in rheumatoid arthritis and in ankylosing spondylarthritis.

Such cases with bulbar disturbances would particularly justify cervico-occipital arthrodesis after reduction and decompression.

Disturbances in sphincter control are most often mild. Hence, they often pass unoticed but should be carefully looked for since they are valuable for the diagnosis. By depriving the bladder of central control, medullary lesions tend to manifest the purely reflex function with incontinence and sudden urination. When the clinical picture is consistent with acute lesion of the spinal cord, the occurrence of reflex urination is preceded by a retention phase corresponding to transient sideration of the spinal reflexes.

Several authors point out the importance of *trophic lesions* but it is almost impossible to know if these lesions are secondary to those of the cervico-occipital joint unless they accompany a major neurological syndrome, e.g., quadriplegia. Most of the time the lesions are confused with those of rheumatoid disease, which also involves the dermo-epidermic cutaneous tissues, the bone tissue, and the muscular tissue. In particular, amyotrophy may be of iatrogenic origin.

An appreciation of the *development of the neurologic manifestations,* though difficult, is of primary importance. The choice between treatment and surgery largely depends on the existence of neurological signs and their development. If it is difficult to affirm the presence of objective neurological involvement, it is even more difficult to appreciate its aggravation, the more so in that some cases may present regressive neurological changes. The important series of Conlon et al. [75] in which no significant neurological manifestation had been recorded at the beginning, showed none after a six-year follow-up (Isdale and Conlon [182]). Ickovic [181] distinguishes major, mean, and minor manifestations.

Concerning the chronology of radiological and clinical features, different factors should be taken into account: on one hand, the delay between the time of occurrence of neurological signs and, on the other, the evolution of the neurological changes from the time of their occurrence on, as we shall see below.

When there are major manifestations atlantoaxial subluxation is readily diagnosed, provided the possibility of such lesions is no longer ignored. Discrete signs, however, should always lead to a search for a cervico-occipital joint lesion. Some studies, Ickovic's for instance, report a delay of 4 years between the occurrence of neurological signs and the time when the diagnosis is made. As a rule, when neurological symptoms are present, they aggravate. In our opinion, the existence of even minor signs, when they are definitely correlated with subluxation, should make one consider surgery.

As a matter of fact, in their 6-year follow-up study of 313 patients Isdale and Conlon [182] did not record any deaths due to neurological complications. But then, their study was mainly radiological with no neurological data presented.

In our opinion, a patient complaining of vague motor or sensory disturbances should not be left to develop quadriplegia, just as a patient with atlantoaxial subluxation should not be left to run the risk of sudden death. However, the age and functional capacity of the patient should be taken into account. This problem will be dealt with in detail in the chapter about treatment.

The determination of the exact *incidence of neurologic manifestations in atlantoaxial subluxations* is difficult, owing to the number of variable factors. In practice, it is impossible to determine the percentage of motor, sensory, or sphincter disturbances, and the type of neurological lesion with regard to the type of subluxation. In the series of rheumatoid arthritis and/or ankylosing spondylarthritis, the selection of cases was done differently. Some did it with regard to the presence or absence of evocative signs, while others took patients in whom the severity of the disease made hospitalization compulsory. Finally, others took groups of patients in whom the severity of the disease was not taken into account. Furthermore, the great variability in the interpretation of the neurological signs intervenes. Our bibliographic study showed considerable differences in the series. Thus, Isdale and Conlon found 84 subluxations without any neurological manifestations among 333 cases of rheumatoid arthritis. Conversely, Stevens studied 100 cases and found 36 subluxations of which 24 had neurological changes. If we add our 250 cases to the largest of these series, we find about 8% of subluxations with neurological manifestations. This figure can be considered minimal.

According to Sharp and Purser [324] it seems that in ankylosing spondylarthritis subluxations are less frequent whereas neurological complications are more so. According to these authors, the usually widespread involvement of the cervical spine in ankylosing spondylarthritis would not allow the nervous structures to adapt as well as with rheumatoid arthritis. It is still not verified whether there is any relationship between the degree of atlantoaxial subluxation and the presence of neurological signs, and if so, the severity of such signs. We shall consider below the critical views about the radiological technique for measuring the subluxation (Part 5, Chapter 5). In any case, this measurement concerns only the bony parts without taking into account the soft parts which could also cause compression. Moreover, the different studies did not make any distinction between anteroposterior atlantoaxial subluxation and upward luxation of the odontoid process, the latter being known only lately. Ickovic [181] and others distinguish subluxations of 5 mm and over 5 mm. This distinction is obviously artificial. Ickovic notes that 89% of the major neurological manifestations are seen in severe atlantoaxial subluxations, whether these are reducible or not. The remaining 11% show that there is no parallelism between the severity of the neurological signs and that of subluxation. As we already pointed out, factors other than bony ones may play a part.

In Stevens' series, 17 of the 36 atlantoaxial subluxations with neurological signs measured between 2 and 5 mm, i.e., about 50%. A similar percentage has been found in other series.

To conclude, we could say schematically that any atlantoaxial subluxation should undergo, at least once a year, a systematic neurologic examination; and that in the case of manifestation of neurological signs, surgery should be considered.

Part 5 Radiology in Rheumatoid Arthritis

Chapter 1 Rarefaction of Bone

Pathological rarefaction of bone in rheumatoid arthritis is not specific for the cervico-occipital joint, since it may involve the whole spine. However, diminution in bone density at this level makes radiodiagnosis particularly difficult. On plain X-rays and even more on tomograms, the outlines of the bones and especially of the odontoid process are hardly visible (Fig. 27). Hypertranslucency of the bones may be so marked as to resemble lysis.

Bone rarefaction, which favors the collapse of the lateral masses of the atlas and fractures of the odontoid process, is considered by some authors to be a cause of secondary basilar invagination (Part 5, Chapter 6). The explanation for the occurrence of this disorder in rheumatoid arthritis is not yet known. The more two varieties of skeletal involvement exist, the more frequently one encounters osteoporosis and the more rarely osteomalacia.

I. Osteoporosis

The relatively high frequency of generalized osteoporosis in rheumatoid arthritis has long been reported. Studies on this subject, however, have multiplied only since the introduction of corticosteroids as a treatment. If the different authors seem to agree about the features of bone rarefaction, they seem to have divergent opinions as regards the respective role of its etiological factors. In 1967, G. Vignon et al. [372] published a study of 281 cases of rheumatoid arthritis and pointed out four factors causing generalized osteoporosis in rheumatoid arthritis.

1. The rheumatic inflammatory process seems to play a role since osteoporosis is the more frequent according to the severity of the arthritis. However, the reason remains hard to explain. According to Ansell and Bywaters [7] it is the inhibition of calcification due to rheumatism. Others incriminate hypercalciuria caused by the disease, but since a usually diminished calciuria exists, this latter mechanism seems very unlikely. Polyarthritis can aggravate hormonal disequilibrium already favored by age and hormone therapy. Perhaps rheumatismal nodules can cause osteolytic vertebral lesions responsible for vertebral collapse.

Besides generalized osteoporosis, there exists also a focalized type of the disorder limited to the surrounding zone of the inflamed articulations and proportional in severity to that of the inflammatory process. Moreover, the bone scan shows an increase of the calcium turnover at the level of the involved articulations (Part 5, Chapter 6).

2. Immobilization may intervene and among Vignon's patients the rate of bedridden persons is 20 out of 79. Immobilization favors demineralization by suppressing the stimulus of the activity of the osteoblasts and by increasing osteolysis. For instance, immobilization of an articulation by ankylosis leads to a more severe osteoporosis at this level.

3. Corticotherapy, a priori, takes a prominent part since osteoporosis being a symptom of Cushing's disease, corticoids favor its progress by slowing down the anabolism of proteins, inhibiting the osteoblasts, and, on the other hand, by reducing intestinal calcium absorption. According to Vignon, the role of corticotherapy is certain but restricted. It increases the frequency of osteoporosis in males and augments its severity in both sexes, thus multiplying the fractures. But it is not an indisputable factor because it has no effect on the frequency of the disease in females.

4. Senile and pre-senile involution seems to play a major role. It could, however, not account for everything since osteoporosis is also encountered in juvenile polyarthritis.

To conclude, we estimate on the basis of our experience that generalized osteoporosis in rheumatoid arthritis is an osteoporosis of pre-senile or senile involution, aggravated by the inflammatory process, immobilization, and corticotherapy, although it is quite difficult to define the degree of bone rarefaction on X-rays. However, taking into account this roentgenologic uncertainty, more than 50% of our cases present significant bone rarefaction (Fig. 5). As far as possible, and in view of the therapeutic indication, we always prefer to ascertain this diagnosis by biopsy (Fig. 6). The seductive hypothesis of an autoimmune systemic mechanism remains to be proved. Conversely, localized osteoporosis in the neighborhood of the involved joints is directly related to the inflammatory process and its severity. Local changes are also mainly various forms of bone tissue loss: from microcysts and erosion to osteonecrosis and massive osteolysis.

II. Osteomalacia

This is another type of skeletal remodeling, which may be encountered in rheumatoid arthritis. From a radiological point of view, we never saw pure osteomalacia in the cervico-occipital region, and especially no cases with pseudofractures or Looser-Milkmann stripes.

Osteomalacia is very rarely isolated, but is usually associated with osteoporotic lesions, thus realizing a mixed syndrome, e.g., osteoporomalacia.

In osteomalacia there is at once a phosphocalcium deficiency caused by diminution of intestinal absorption and increased elimination caused by lesions in the renal tubules. Vitamin D deficiency is usually necessary for osteomalacia to occur. This deficiency can be due to a lack of sun exposure, especially in the case of bedridden patients.

To illustrate the problem of bone rarefaction, we report on three cases in which bone biopsy showed marked osteoporosis in two and osteomalacia in the third (Dirheimer [100]). However, there was no roentgenologic evidence of bone rarefaction in any of the three cases. Conversely, case No. 2 (Fig. 31 d) showed hyperostosis in the area of the odontoid process and of the anterior arch of the atlas.

L... Marie, a 53-year-old female, suffered for 15 years from classical seropositive rheumatoid polyarthritis grade 3, and had never been treated with steroids.
Iliac crest biopsy. Decalcified sample (biopsy report: Prof. P. Meunier, Laboratoire d'histodynamique osseuse, Lyon). Between two cortices of 1560 and 1250 µm thickness, rarefaction of the spongy bone. The trabecular volume was 12.3% (normal values at the same age: 19.9 ± 3.6). Absence of trabecular hyperosteoclastosis. The trabecular osteoclastic resorption

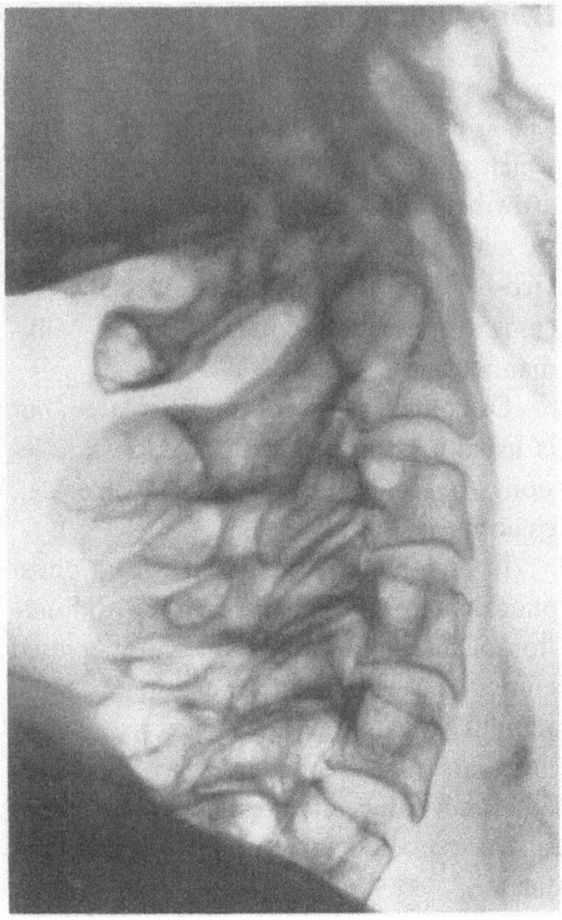

Fig. 5. A 60-year-old female with marked vertebral osteoporosis and numerous vertebral collapses in the thoracic and lumbar spine. Bone biopsy shows a very low absolute trabecular bone volume (11.5%), whereas the osteoid volume is normal (0.29%). In the cervical spine, note hypertranslucent vertebrae and trabecular bone rarefaction; contours of the vertebrae are more clearly outlined than normally. Cervical hyperlordosis compensates marked dorsal kyphosis secondary to vertebral collapse

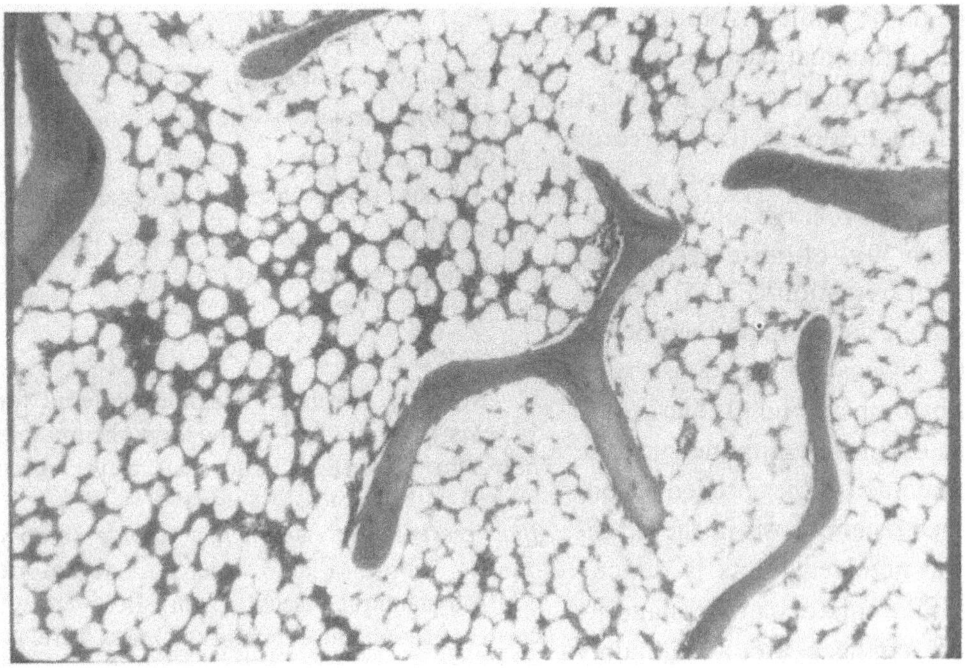

Fig. 6. Iliac crest biopsy in a case of osteoporosis secondary to corticosteroids. Ribbon-shaped, very narrow and short bone trabeculae in a marrow undergoing marked adipose involution. (Courtesy of P. Meunier, Lyon)

surfaces were within normal limits, i.e. 3.2% (3.6 ±1.1). Some large endohaversian osteoclastic foci. The periosteocytic lacunae were widened and measured 59.1 μm² (50.7 ±5.5). The marrow underwent adipose involution and the volume of adipose tissue in the marrow was 76.2%.

Undecalcified sample: Between the two cortices of normal thickness (720 and 500 μm), the rarefaction of the trabecular bone seems milder than on the decalcified fragment. The resorption surfaces are, at 4.5%, at the upper limit of the normal values (3.6 ± 1.1).

The osteoid volume is normal: 2.8% (3.2 ± 1.7) as well as the osteoid surfaces: 18.1% (13.5 ± 6.5).

These findings are consistent with pure osteoporosis with slightly increased resorption parameters.

J... Lucie, a 50-year-old female with classical seropositive grade 3 rheumatoid polyarthritis for 14 years. This patient had been treated with prednisone (10–15 mg) for 6 years (Fig. 31 d). *Iliac crest biopsy* (decalcified sample). Very thick cortex (2300 μm) with rare and discontinuous trabeculae. The trabecular volume was low with regard to the age: 13.9% (19.9 ± 3.6). Normal resorption surfaces with 4.1%. Normal periostic lacunae; 51.8% (50.6 ±5.2). The volume of adipose tissue in the marrow was normal: 43%. Possible hyperosteoidosis.

Conclusion: osteoporosis.

Undecalcified sample: Complete bioptic cylinder; well-preserved structure outlined by thick and compact cortices (1600 and 900 μm). Obvious atrophy of cancellous bone. The trabecular bone volume is 11.1%, which is low with regard to the age (19.9 ± 3.6). Osteoid volume normal: 1.4%. Osteoid surfaces normal: 4.3%. The rate of calcification is readily measurable with fluorescent light thanks to double marking with tetracycline. It is normal at 1.14 μm per day in the compact bone and lowered to 0.80 μm per day in the cancellous bone.

Conclusion: pure osteoporosis with elective inertia of the osteoblastic apposition at the level of the cancellous bone.

Woe... Marguerite, 54-year-old female. Seronegative definite polyarthritis for $3^1/_2$ years. Never treated with steroids.
Iliac creast biopsy (undecalcified sample). The cylinder was incomplete and comprised a very thin and fractured cortex 300 μm thick. The structure of the spongy bone seemed poorly preserved. The trabecular bone volume could not be measured, but there seemed to be rarefaction of the trabeculae.

The relative osteoid volume was markedly increased – 8% (1.6 ± 0.7 for same age and sex). The osteoid surfaces were increased to 26% (8.6 ± 3.9). The thickness index of the osteoid apposition was increased to 30 (18.5 ± 2.5).

Conclusion: definite osteomalacia on a probably overall rarefied bone.

Chapter 2 Articular Changes: Arthritis

Classically, there are no radiological changes at the very onset of rheumatoid arthritis. At best, in the joints of the limbs, a slight widening of the articular interspace is visible, consistent with tumefaction of the soft parts and hypertrophy of the synovia. We have never observed these features in the atlanto-occipital or atlantoaxial joints. We shall deal separately (Part 5, Chapter 5) with the problem of the atlanto-odontoid joint. Adjacent decalcification and narrowing of the interspace due to destruction of cartilage occurs more or less quickly. The narrowing of an interspace is readily recognizable provided correct radiographic technique has been utilized, i.e., positioning of the head, beam direction, projection.

When narrowing of the interspace is evident, it is useful to assess whether it is acquired or congenital. Wackenheim [380] points out that narrowing of the atlanto-condylar interspace is seen in cases with a tendency to occipitalization of the atlas or in anomalies accompanied by narrowing of all interspaces in the cervico-occipital region.

All articular interspaces may be involved, more or less symmetrically: the occipitoatlantal joint (Figs. 7–10, 14, 21, 23, 33, 34, 35, 62), the atlantoaxial joint (Figs. 9, 10, 23, 39, 49), and the anterior atlanto-odontoid joint, the narrowing of which is more rare and then, usually, of late occurrence (Figs. 13, 61, 81).

Van Kerckhove [365] studied the atlantoaxial joint in 606 patients with rheumatoid arthritis and in 30 cases be discovered articular changes, although in only 16 of them was there isolated narrowing of the articular interspace. In the other 14, he noted associated bone lesions. In 2 cases atlantoaxial arthritis was the primary location of the disease (1 case of seronegative rheumatoid arthritis and 1 case of juvenile polyarthritis). According to this author, there is a correlation between involvement of the atlantoaxial joint and the state of the other joints in general. Serre et al. [316] studied the atlanto-occipital articulations in 30 of their 59 patients and the atlantoaxial articulations in 40. In the cases without atlantoaxial subluxation, they found atlanto-occipital arthritis in 3 cases out of 15, in 1 bilaterally, atlantoaxial arthritis in 7 of 23 cases. Among the latter 7 cases, 3 had bilateral and 4 unilateral arthritis. Among the 15 cases without subluxation, atlanto-occipital arthritis was present in 6 cases of which 4 were bilateral, and inferior arthritis in 10 cases, of which 4 were bilateral. In our material we found twice as many cases with atlanto-occipital arthritis as with atlantoaxial arthritis. The number of unilateral involvements is roughly the same as that of bilateral.

Like Serre et al., we record twice as much arthritis in cases with atlantoaxial subluxation as in cases without. Moreover, there are always one or several cases of arthritis in our cases with upward atlantoaxial subluxation (see Part 5, Chapter 5).

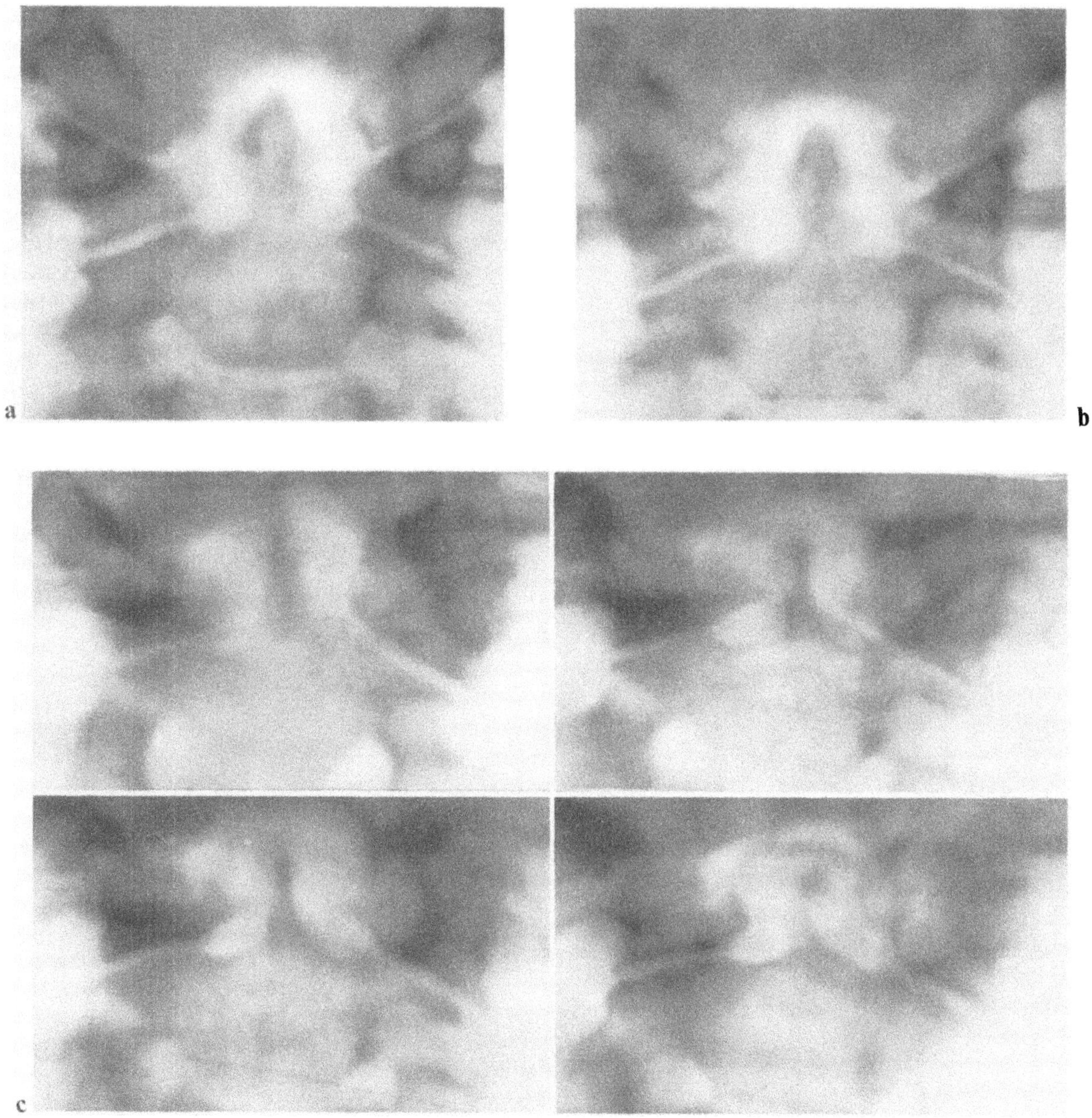

Fig. 7. **(a)** X-rays taken on the 9-5-72 in a patient with rheumatoid arthritis. Slight narrowing of right occipitoatlantal interspace with sclerosis of the lateral mass of the atlas and condyles. **(b)** X-rays taken on the 3-29-73 in the same patient. The previous anomalies are more prononced. Erosions of the base of the odontoid process—were already present 6 months ago (a)—are now clearly visible. **(c)** X-rays taken on 11-26-74 in the same patient. Lateral subluxation of the atlas towards the left and collapse of its right lateral mass. The left occipitoatlantal joint is also involved. Marked lysis of odontoid process

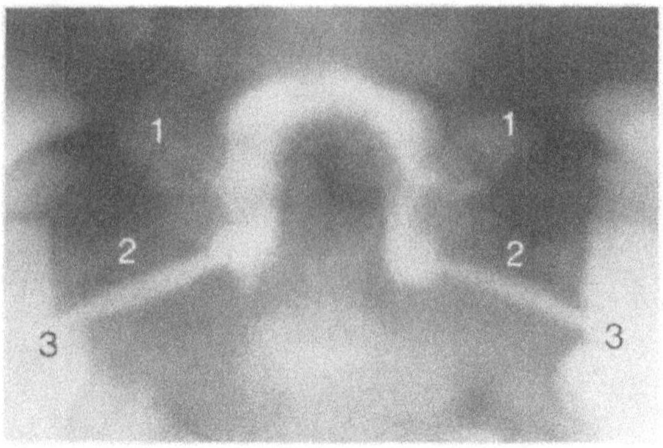

Fig. 8. Bilaterally destroyed articular surfaces of occipitoatlantal joint *(1)* with undamaged atlantoaxial joints *(2)*. Note, however, moderate lateral atlantoaxial subluxation towards the left *(3)*

a
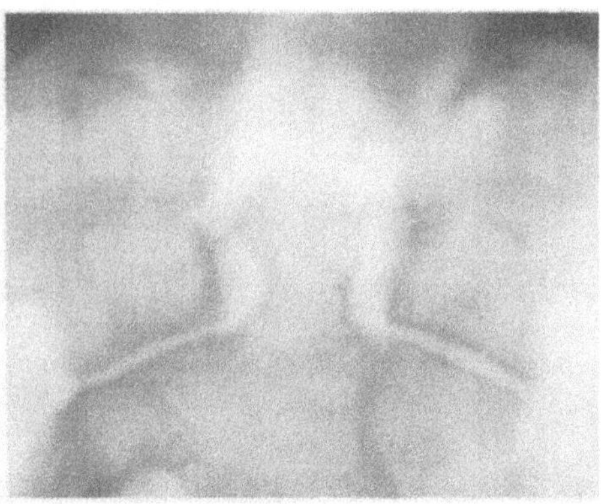

Fig. 9a and b. Legend see opposite page

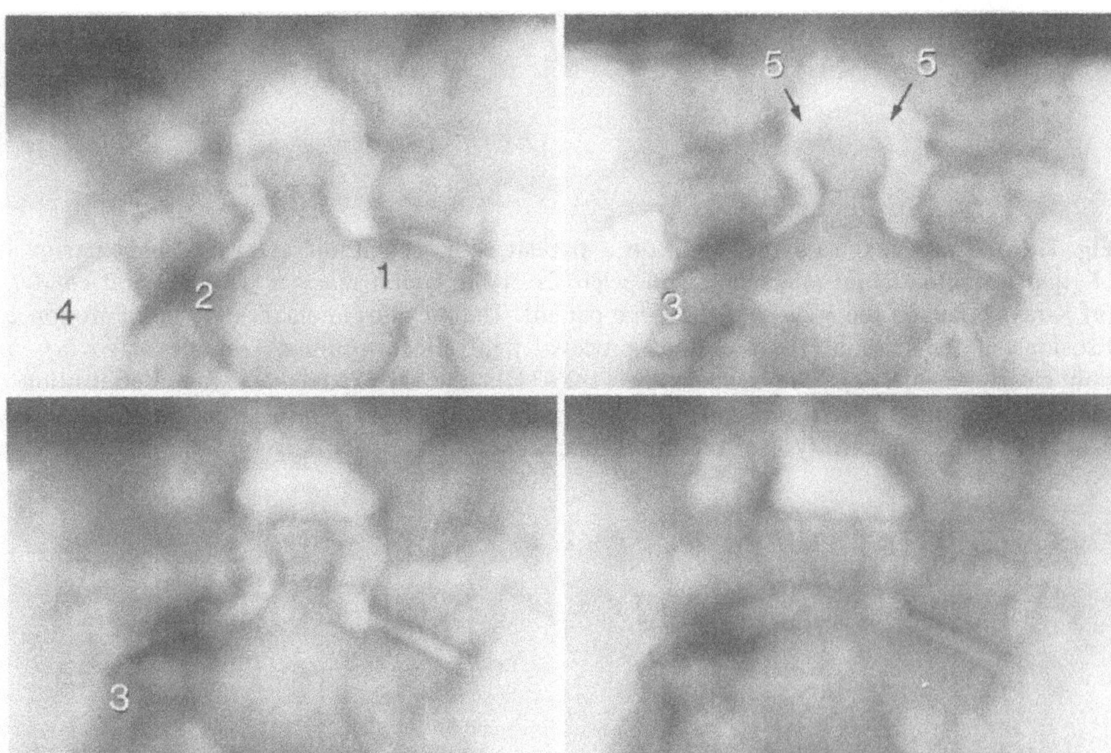

b

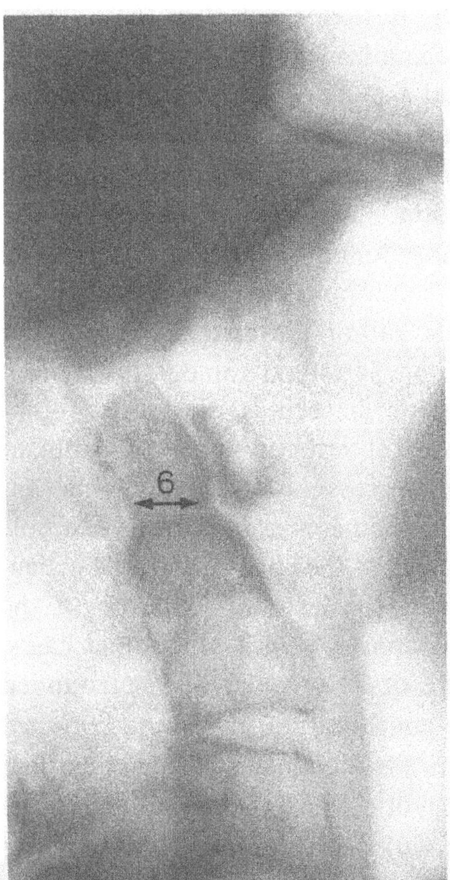

b

Fig. 9a and b. Bilateral atlantoaxial arthritis in a case of advanced bilateral occipitoatlantal arthritis. **(a)** 1972: narrowing of the right and, to a lesser degree, of the left atlantoaxial interspace. **(b)** 1973: multiple lesions. *1* Narrowed left atlantoaxial interspace, *2* Narrowing, erosion, and sclerosis of right atlantoaxial interspace, *3* Translucency of the right superior articular process of the axis, *4* C1/2 rotation subluxation, *5* Erosion of odontoid tip, *6* Anterior and posterior erosion of odontoid process

Chapter 3 Destructive Bone Lesions

(Pseudocysts, Encroachments, Erosions, Destructions, Lysis, and Fractures)

Pseudocysts on the hands and feet are common findings in rheumatoid arthritis. They are rarer in the cervico-occipital region, except perhaps for the odontoid process. Some of the pseudocysts correspond to encroachments seen on frontal views, others are intraosseous cavities. They occur early, are rounded or oval-shaped, and usually multiple and rather small. When they extend, they are poorly outlined and may be surrounded by osteosclerosis when they become coalescent. Small constitutional pseudocysts may be seen in the lateral masses of the atlas but they never have the same blurred aspect with now and then interrupted or condensed margins. Diffuse demineralization and eventual narrowing of the atlanto-occipital or lateral atlantoaxial interspaces are arguments in favor of polyarthritic pseudocysts.

These lesions cause a more or less widespread destruction of the adjacent bone. They are rarely present in the occipital condyles, in the lateral masses of the atlas (Figs. 7, 9–11, 14), upper articular processes of the axis, and even more rarely in the anterior arch of the atlas. Conversely, such formations, sometimes of large size, are often seen to occupy the largest part of the odontoid process (Figs. 19, 66). This major bone lesion exposes the patient to severe complications by collapse of the dens or by progressive destruction of the odontoid process producing atlantoaxial subluxation.

By *encroachment* we mean a small indentation in the margin of the capsulosynovial attachment. Between encroachment and erosion there is only a difference of size, but the demarcation between these two lesions is not otherwise well-defined.

Often poorly outlined while growing, encroachments and pseudocysts may be surrounded by osteosclerosis when they become coalescent. They produce more or less widespread *erosions*. These have preferential sites related to the anatomical disposition of the synovial membranes, i.e. the clivus, the posterior aspect of the anterior arch of the atlas, the tip of the odontoid, the lateral aspects of the odontoid process, sometimes the anterior articular facet of the odontoid and, mainly, the posterior aspect of the odontoid process at the level of the syndesmo-odontoid joint (Fig. 15).

This condition has been described by numerous authors; Martel [223] found it 12 times on 34 lateral tomograms. It is a severe lesion since it is most often associated with anterior atlantoaxial subluxation. All degrees of severity may be encountered. Sometimes it is only a simple accentuation of the concavity of the articular facet at the level of the neck of the odontoid process (Fig. 17). In other cases, it is more or less regular and surrounded by bone condensation and so accentuated as to form a true cupula resulting in marked erosion of the odontoid process (Figs. 18–20). The erosion may be so severe that the odontoid process is entirely rup-

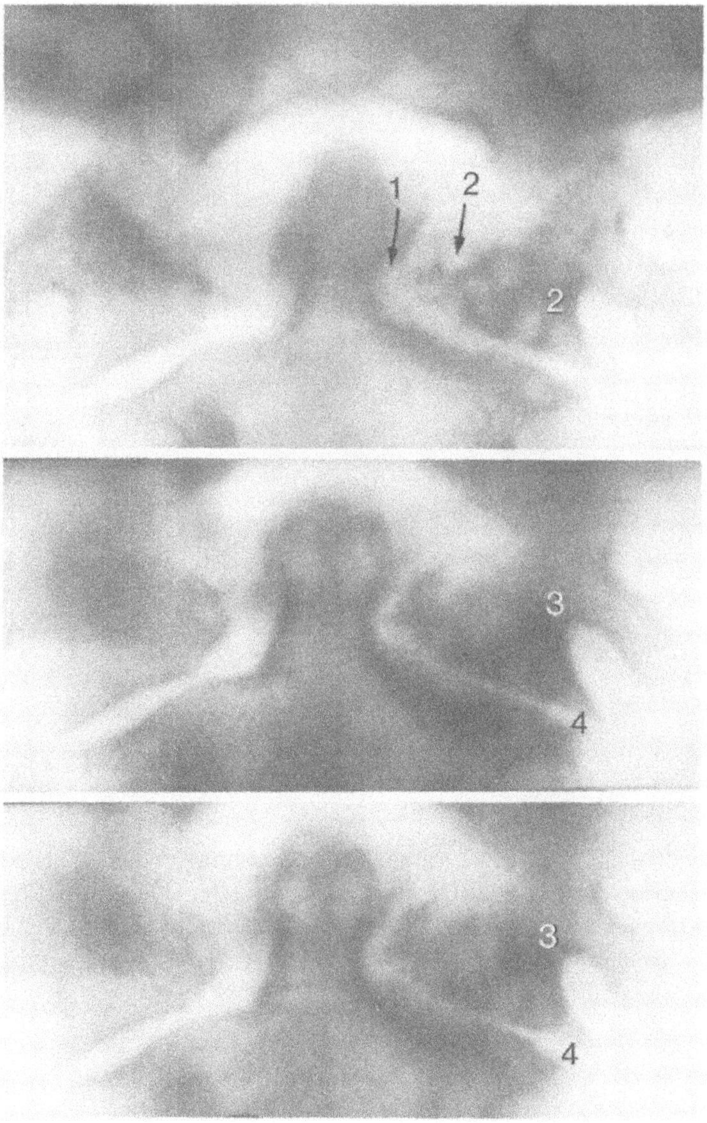

Fig. 10. Multiple lesions in rheumatoid arthritis. *1* Erosion of the base of the odontoid, *2* Numerous erosions in left lateral mass of the atlas, *3* Translucencies of left lateral mass of the atlas, *4* Erosion of left superior articular surface of the axis

tured from its base, resulting in a fracture of the process. Irregular edges suggest that the fracture occurred in an eroded area. According to Martel, this type of lesion is seen in about 1% of cases. The free bone fragment may either ascend above the anterior arch or decrease in size, undergo lysis and disappear. When there is a pre-existent atlantoaxial subluxation, the free fragment does not follow the movements of the odontoid during the functional flexion-extension examination. Fracture of the odontoid process is to be distinguished from a malformation, i.e. absence of fusion of the dens. According to Jung [189] and Wackenheim [380], in case of fracture of the base of the odontoid process, the extension movements of the head usually reduce the fracture, while in densaplasia reduction is effected by flexion of the head. In case of lysis of the free fragment, the differential diagnosis has to be made with regard to congenital absence of the odontoid process.

Moreover, this fracture makes possible a posterior atlantoaxial subluxation (Part 5, Chapter 5).

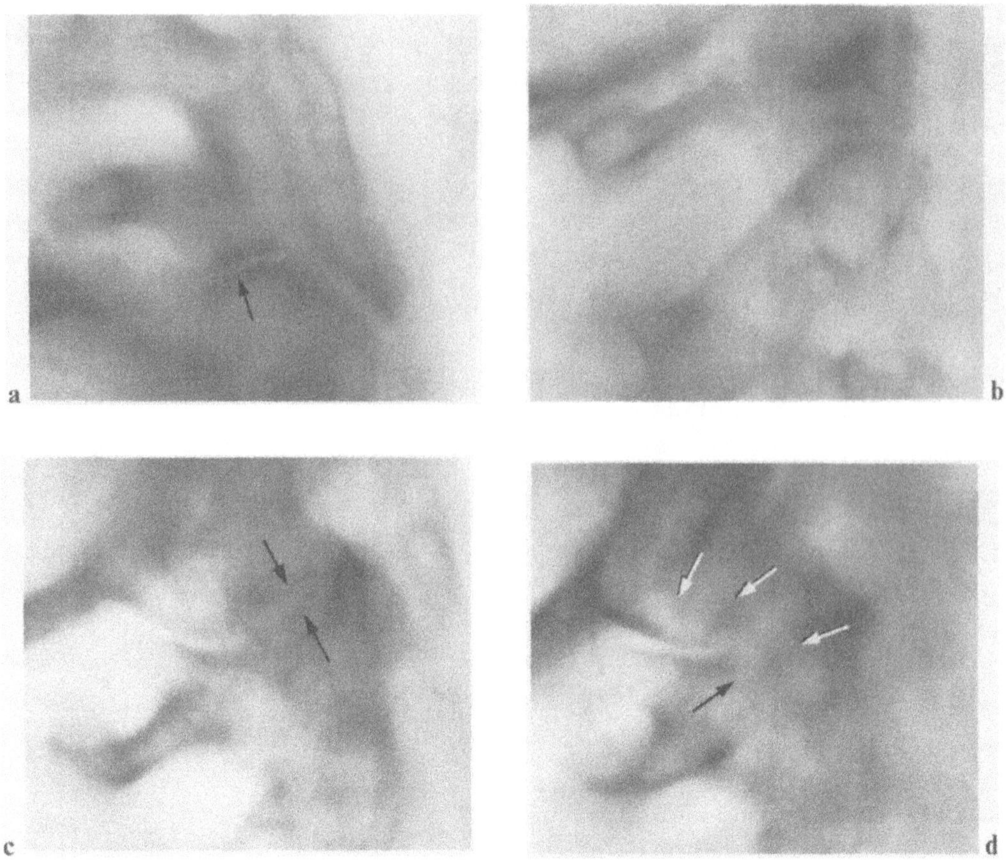

Fig. 11 a–d. Lateral views in arthritis of occipitoatlantal joints. **(a)** Narrowing of the posterior part of interspace, **(b)** Narrowing of entire occipitoatlantal interspace, **(c)** Irregular destruction of articular surfaces, **(d)** Subchondral translucencies

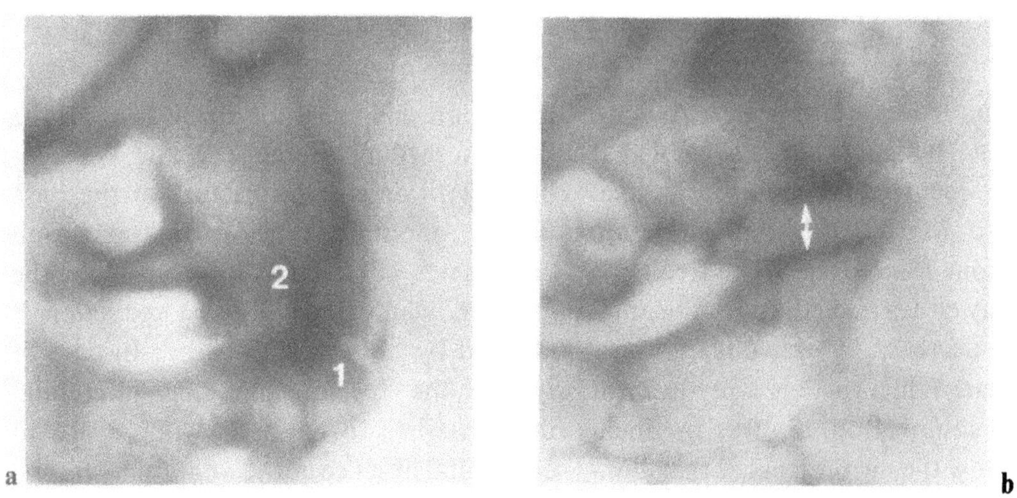

Fig. 12 a and b. Lateral views in arthritis of the atlantoaxial joints in two cases of rheumatoid arthritis. **(a)** Narrowing and sclerosis of the middle part of the interspace *(1)*. Translucencies of a lateral mass of the atlas *(2)*. **(b)** Irregular and widened atlantoaxial interspace

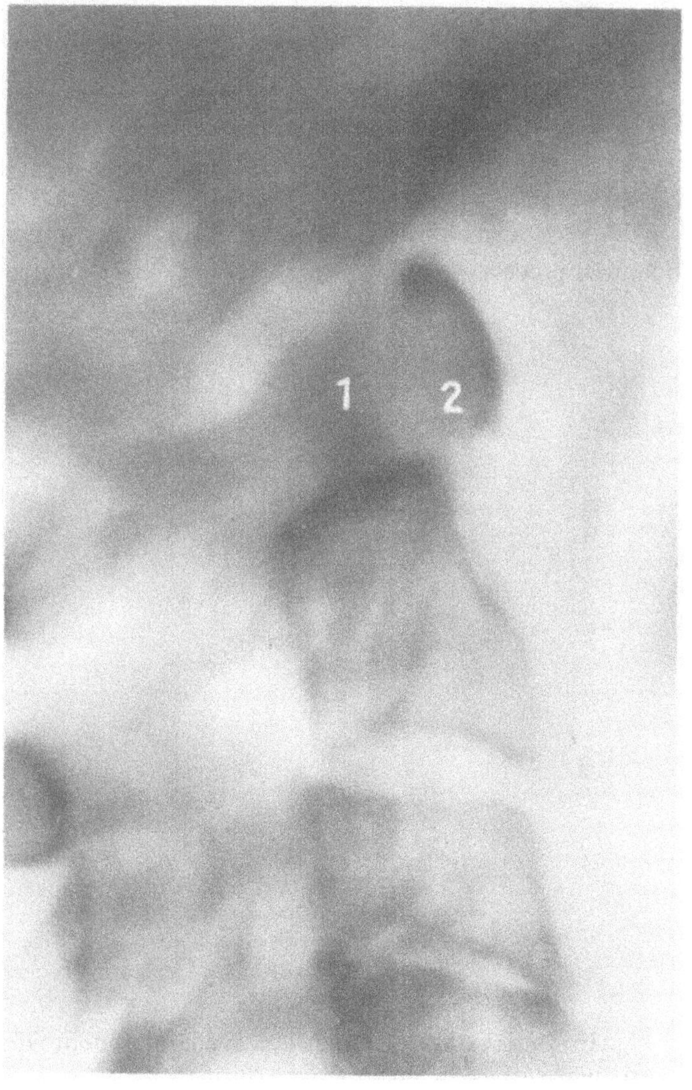

Fig. 13. Osteolysis of the odontoid process *(1)* and of the posterior aspect of the anterior arch of the atlas *(2)* in rheumatoid arthritis

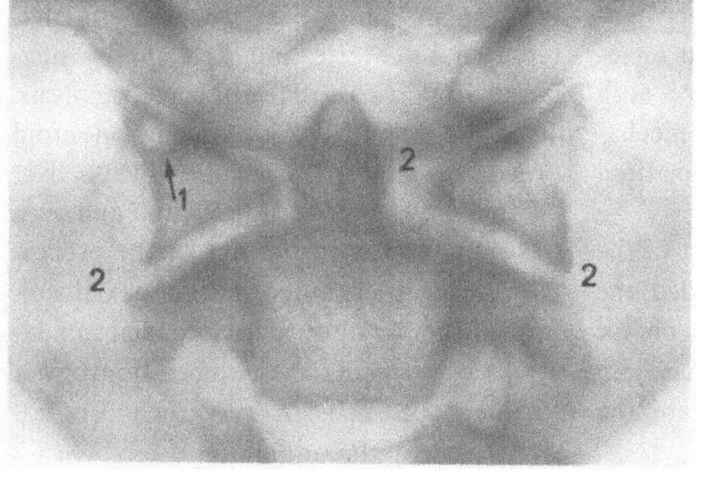

Fig. 14. Translucency with sclerotic borderlines in the right lateral mass of the atlas *(1)*. Atlantoaxial rotation *(2)*

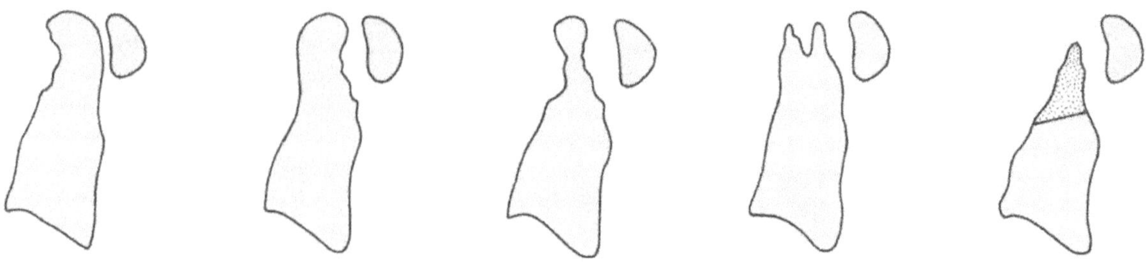

Fig. 15. Various types of erosion of the odontoid process

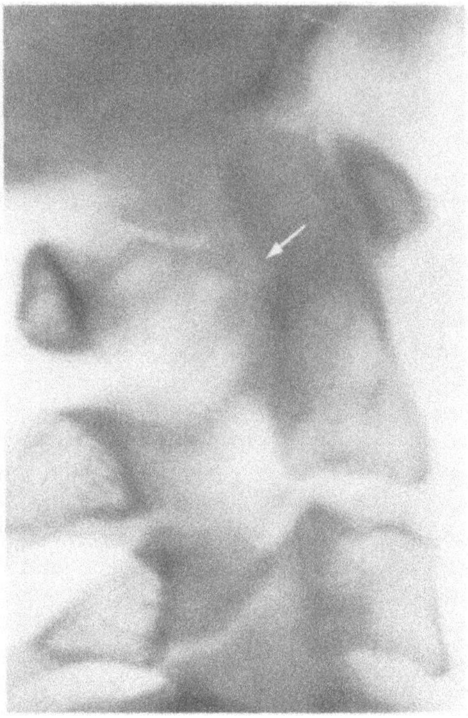

Fig. 16. Initial stage of an eroded syndesmo-odontoid articular surface in rheumatoid arthritis

Erosion of both atlanto-odontoid articular aspects is more rare. When present, the size of the anterior arch of the atlas decreases and its posterior margin becomes blurred (Figs. 13, 20, 81). One could imagine total destruction of the anterior arch and this would account for a second mechanism of posterior atlantoaxial subluxation.

When the anterior articular facet of the odontoid process happens to be eroded, the erosion is always less marked than on the posterior facet. This erosive area may join the posterior one and thus facilitate the fractures (Figs. 9b, 13, 20).

The tip of the odontoid process may also be eroded and progressively destroyed (Figs. 13, 61, 77). The odontoid takes on the "sugar-loaf aspect" similar to that reported by Marie and Leri in the phalanges in polyarthritis with acro-osteolysis. The total height of the axis and odontoid process, which is normally always over 40 mm, may be reduced to 35 mm and even less. Diminution in the size of the process plays a role in the anterior atlantoaxial subluxation and in upward atlantoaxial subluxations by reducing the compression power of this bone. Erosion may then progressively destroy the odontoid.

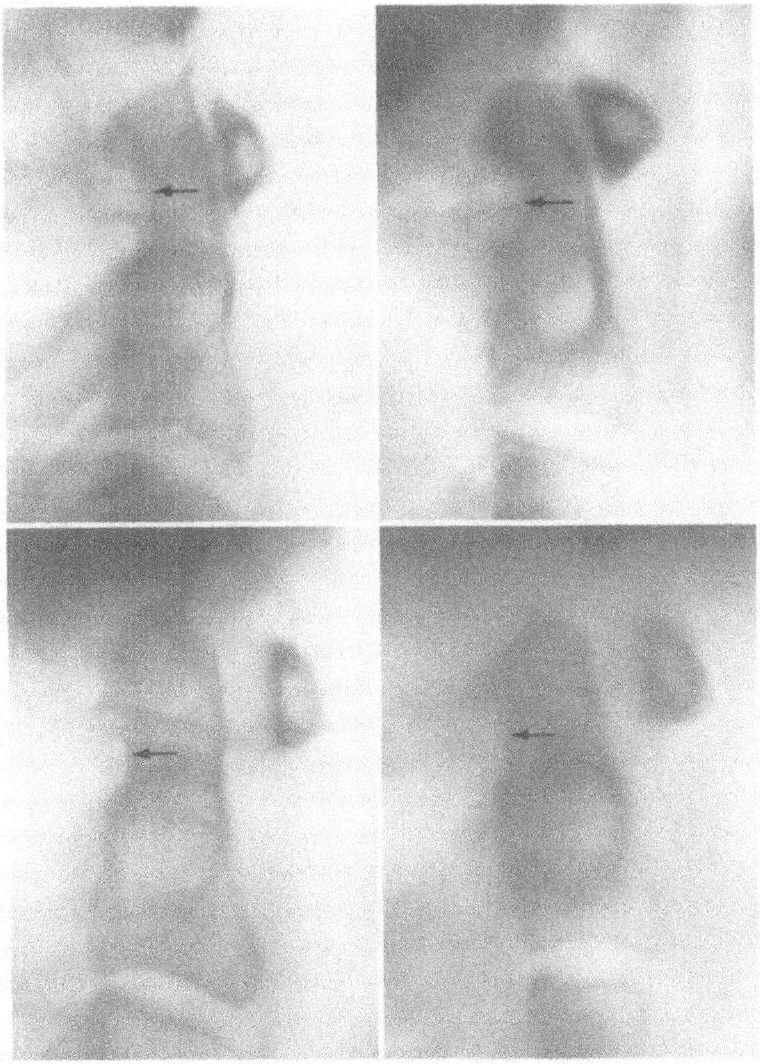

Fig. 17. Four types of erosion of posterior aspect of the odontoid, with more or less accentuated cupula. These lesions of the syndesmo-odontoid joint, and consequently of the transverse ligament, may be responsible for anterior atlantoaxial subluxation *(two bottom figures)*

Erosion and destruction of the odontoid may sometimes be visualized on frontal X-rays. The size of the odontoid is diminished transversely as well as in height and this condition may be called "atrophy of the dens" (Figs. 7, 21, 22, 49).

We have already reported the possible existence of a bursa between the tip of the dens and the clivus. This bursa can be a localization of synovitis and then the area of the basion is destroyed, causing widening of the foramen magnum. Martel systematically measured Boogard's angle and found it significantly increased. As concerns our series of cases, the inferior clivus was sometimes hardly visible, i.e. demineralized, but we never found erosion in this area.

In the chapter dealing with arthritis, we mentioned the possibility of destructions occurring in the occipitoatlantal and atlantoaxial joints. There may be partial *destruction* or *lysis* of the bone parts entailing their compression or collapse. The lateral mass of the atlas, the most frequently involved,

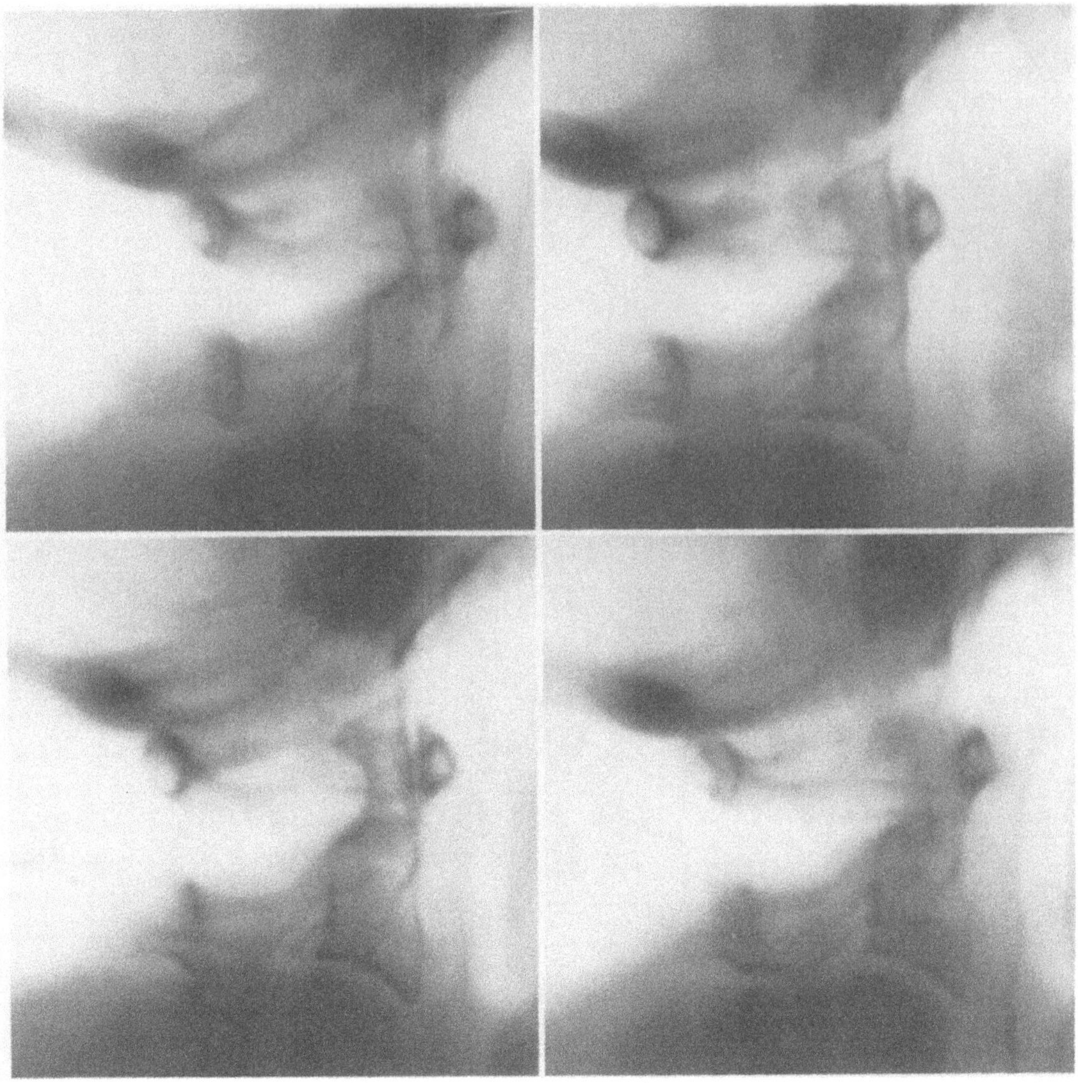

Fig. 18. Different tomographic sections in a case of widespread posterior erosion of the odontoid process in rheumatoid arthritis

may be reduced to a half or even a third of its size, impacted and serrated into the occipital condyle or into the articular surface of the axis. These features are similar to those of fused carpitis, the ultimate state in wrist involvement (Figs. 7–10, 49).

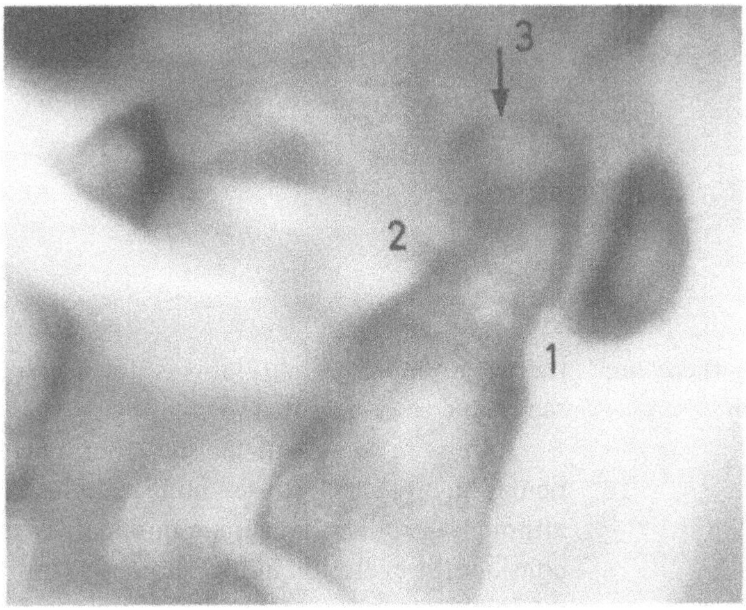

Fig. 19. Multiple lesions of the odontoid process in rheumatoid arthritis. *1* Anterior cupula due to erosion in the synovial region of the anterior atlanto-odontoid joint, *2* Posterior cupula due to erosion in the synovial region of the syndesmo-odontoid joint, *3* Irregular demineralization with apical erosion. Note that clivus is intact

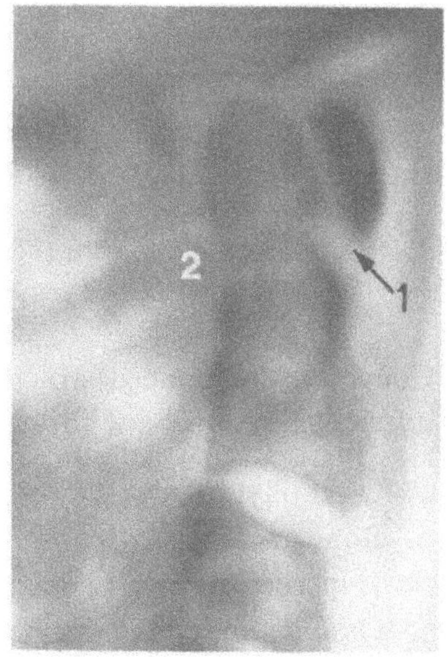

Fig. 20. Erosion of the anterior aspect of the odontoid process *(1)*. On the posterior aspect, irregular mineralization of the corticalis: initial stage of erosion *(2)*

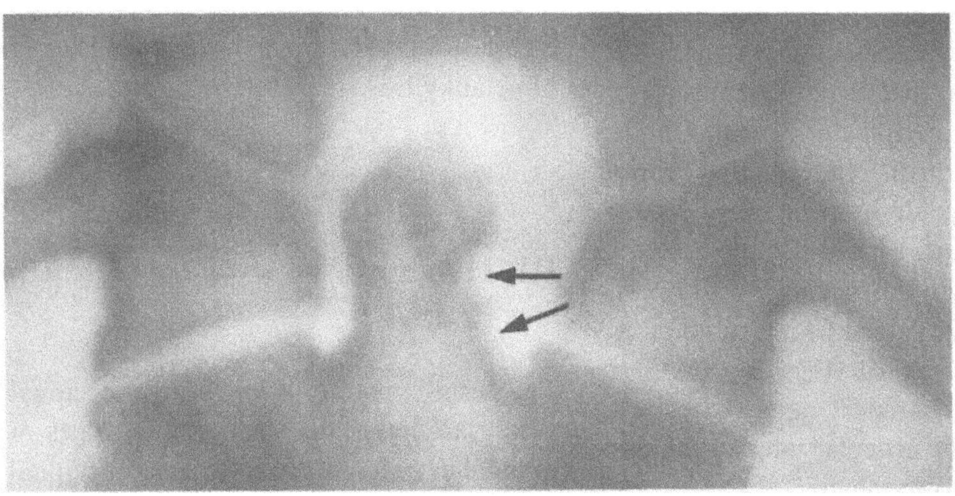

Fig. 21. Erosion of the lateral aspect of the odontoid process in rheumatoid arthritis

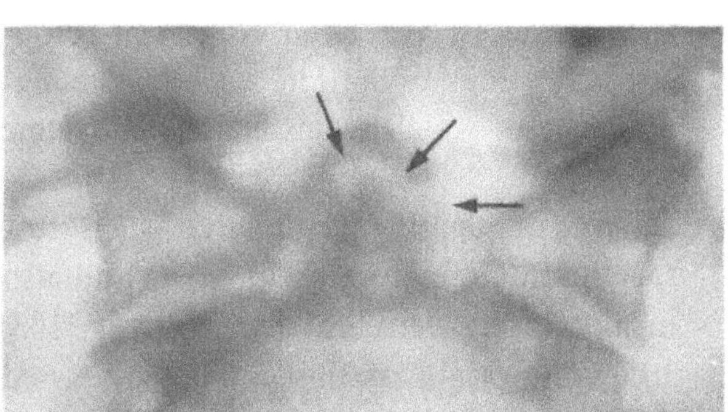

Fig. 22. Widespread destruction of the left part of the odontoid process in rheumatoid arthritis

Chapter 4 Constructive Bone Lesions

Conversely to bone destruction, there are different types of bone formation:

- Osteophytes
- Bone ankylosis
- Hyperostosis
- Ossification of the ligaments
- Ossification of the meninges.

I. Osteophytes

It is well known that osteophytes are rarely found in the peripheral articulations in rheumatoid arthritis. Indeed, they appear in this site only late in the stage of secondary osteoarthritis. This is also the case with the cervico-occipital region. We have seen them in only six cases of long-standing arthritis (up to 25 years) (Figs. 23, 39). Serre et al. [316] also report some cases with narrowing of the articular interspaces, condensation and osteophytes.

II. Bone Ankylosis

True bone ankylosis also is very rare. Sometimes the interspace is not visible, but functional examinations show that a certain degree of mobility is preserved. Even when there is no more mobility, this is not necessarily due to bone ankylosis.

Rarely, in some patients, peripheral articular involvement causes bone ankylosis although the bone changes are minimal. We consider the evolution in the cervico-occipital joints to follow a similar pattern. In the two cases illustrated in Figures 24 and 25, the ossified ligaments are readily visualized as linear opacities, whereas the atlanto-odontoid articular interspace is no longer visible. As we already pointed out, destruction of the condyles, lateral masses of atlas, and axis by arthritis may lead to bone ankylosis.

III. Hyperostosis

The term "manifestation of the occipital vertebra" classically denotes two types of anomalies occurring in the cervico-occipital joints, i.e. anomalies of defect, which shall not be dealt with in this chapter, and anomalies of excess. The latter consist in ectopic ossifications of infinite variety, the significance of which seems exactly the same to us.

We frequently encountered such features in inflammatory rheumatism and also in ankylosing vertebral hyperostosis [103, 105]. The origin of this will be discussed further on.

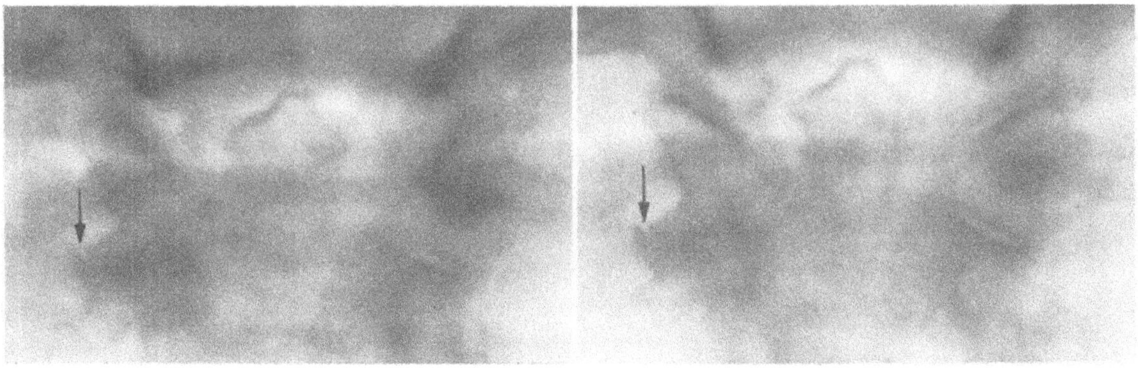

Fig. 23. Advanced stage of non-progressing rheumatoid arthritis and secondary osteoarthritis with osteophytes

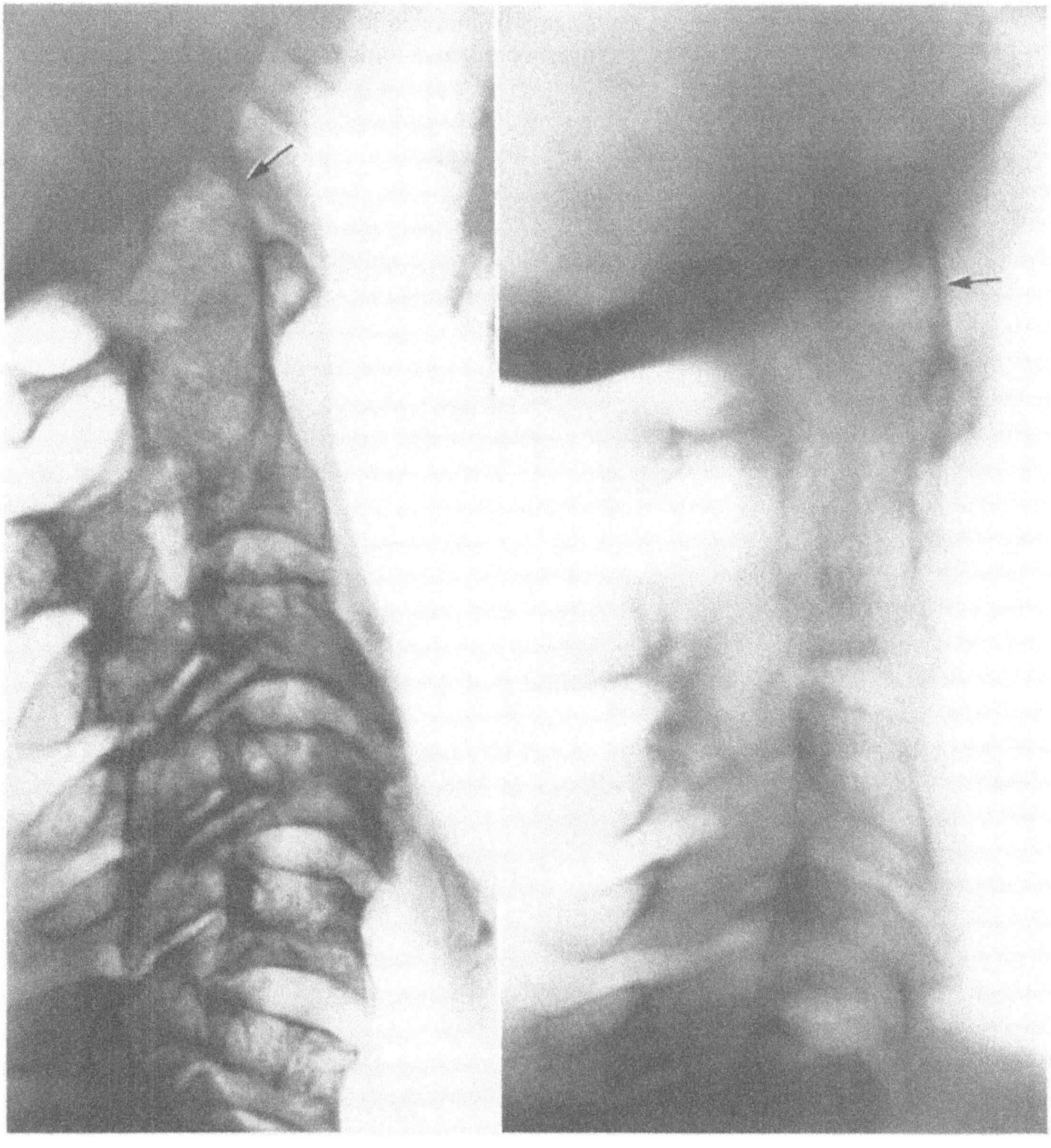

Fig. 24. Calcification or ossification of ligaments in a case of rheumatoid arthritis

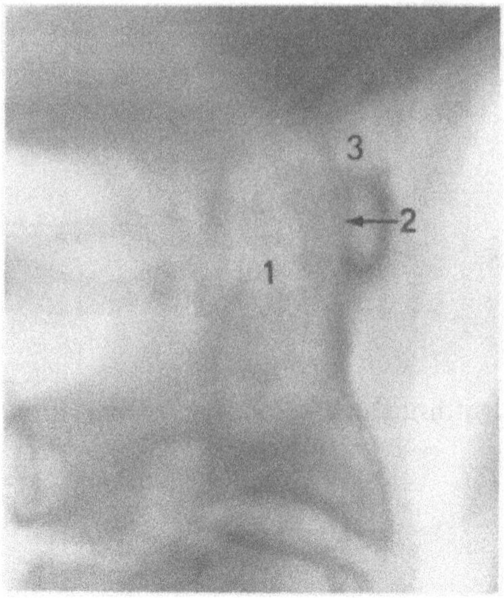

Fig. 25. Rheumatoid arthritis evolving for 25 years. Highly demineralized odontoid process *(1)*, ankylosis of atlantodental joint *(2)*, and ossified ligament *(3)*

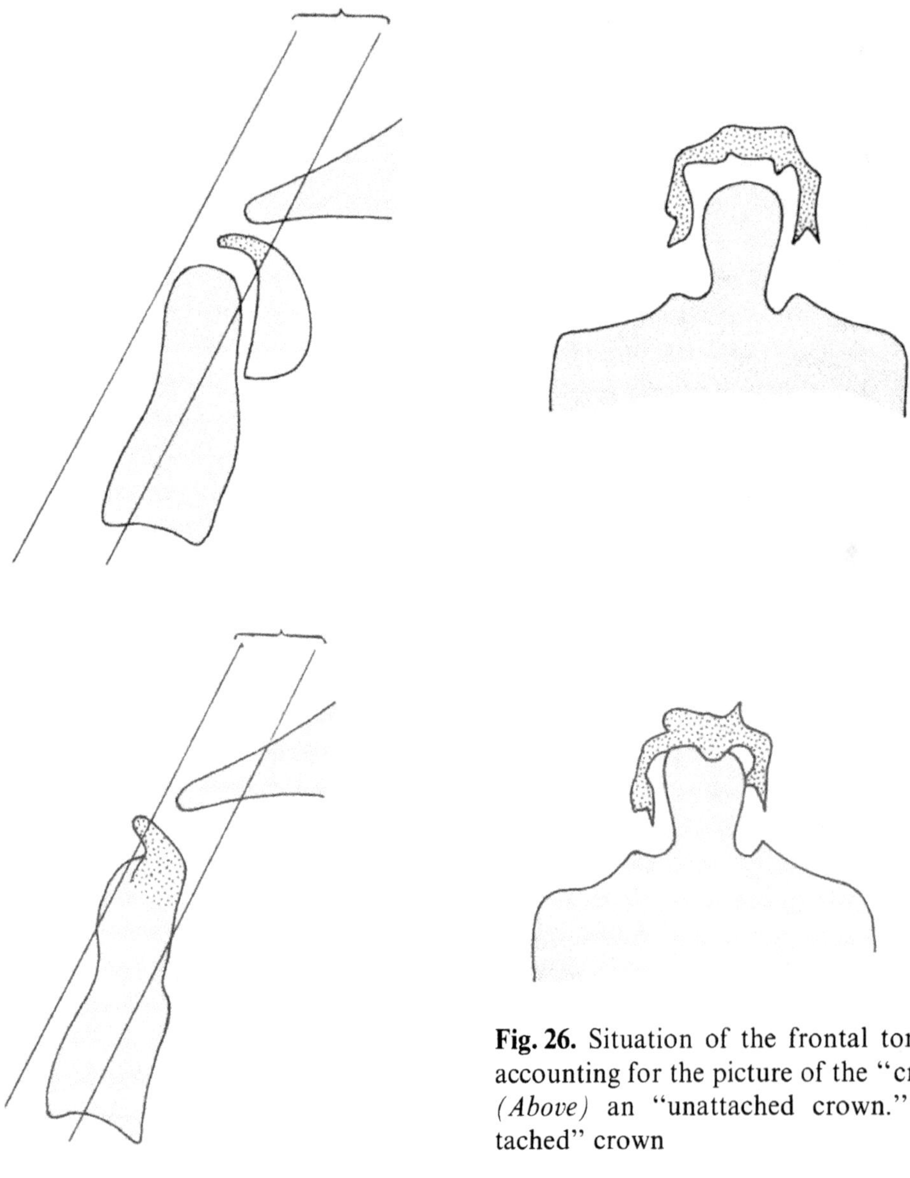

Fig. 26. Situation of the frontal tomographic sections accounting for the picture of the "crowned odontoid." *(Above)* an "unattached crown." *(Below)* an "attached" crown

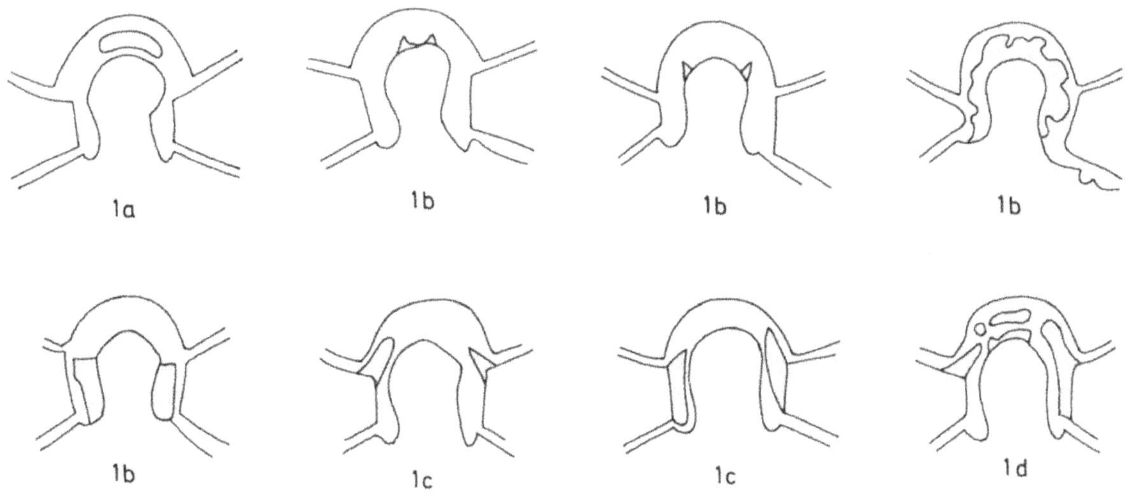

Fig. 27. Different types of hyperostosis in frontal sections of the odontoid process. (See Part 5, Chapt. 4)

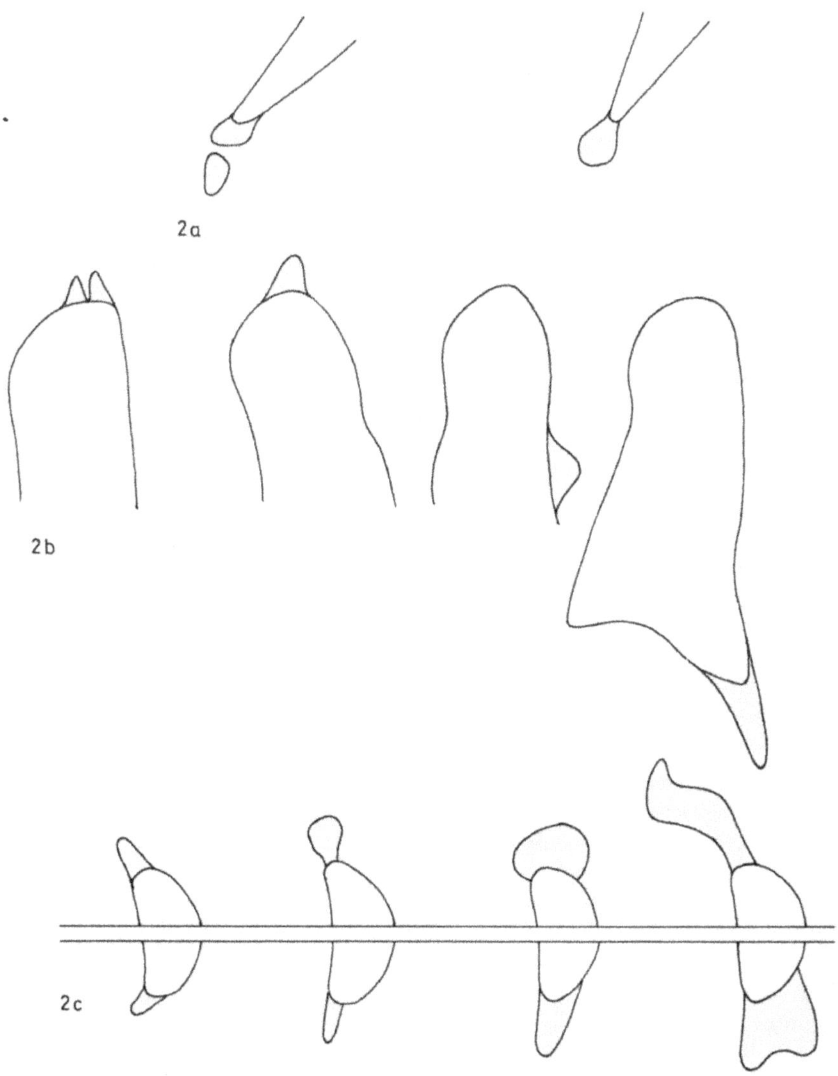

Fig. 28. Different types of hyperostosis in lateral sections. (See Part 5, Chapt. 4)

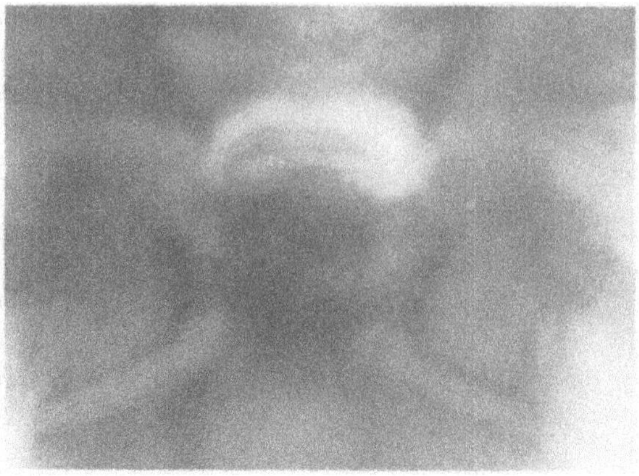

Fig. 29. "Crowned odontoid process" in rheumatoid arthritis. Note the dense odontoid (shining odontoid) and its blurred borders

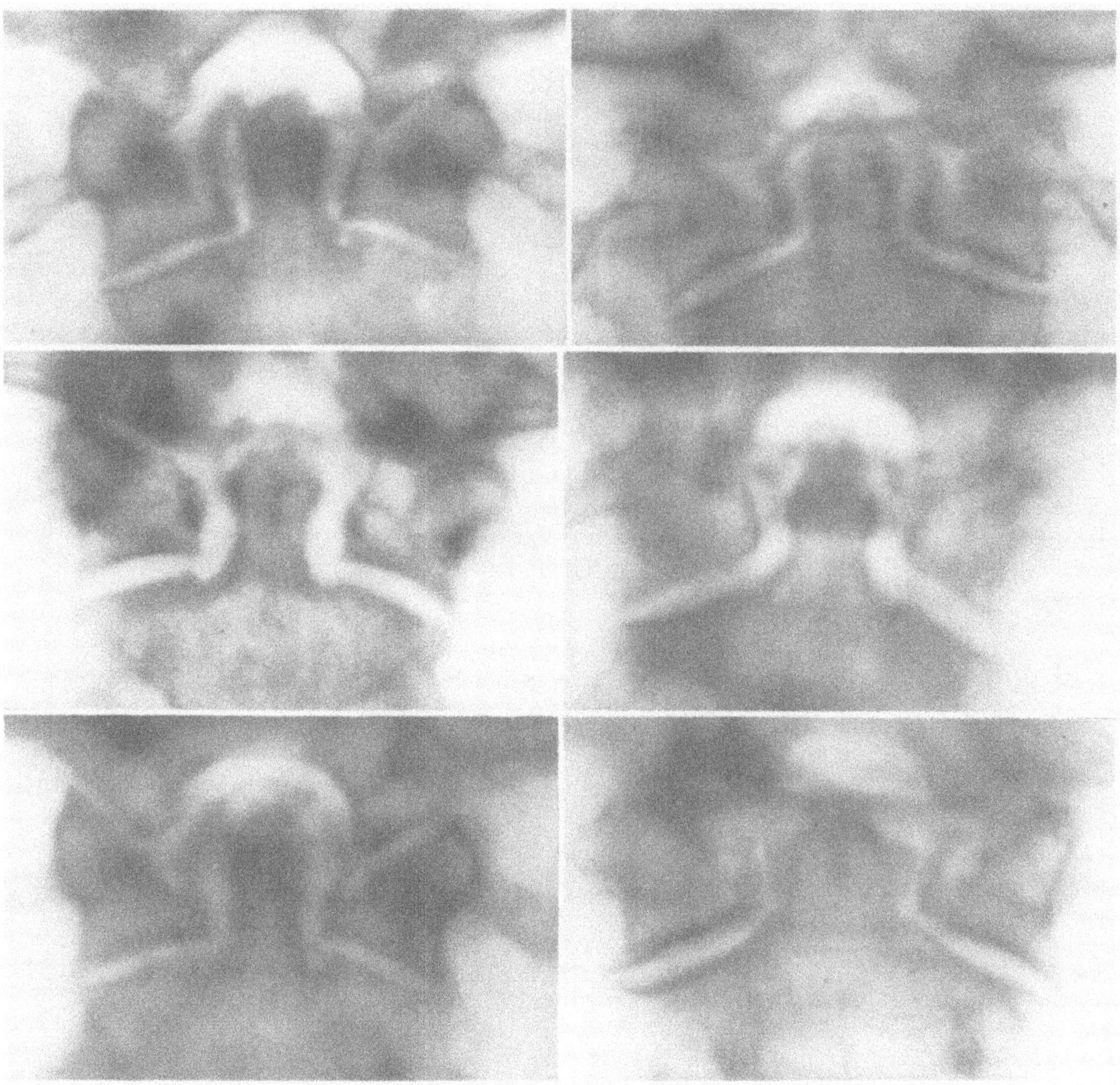

Fig. 30. Different types of hyperostosis in rheumatoid arthritis. Frontal views at the level of the odontoid process

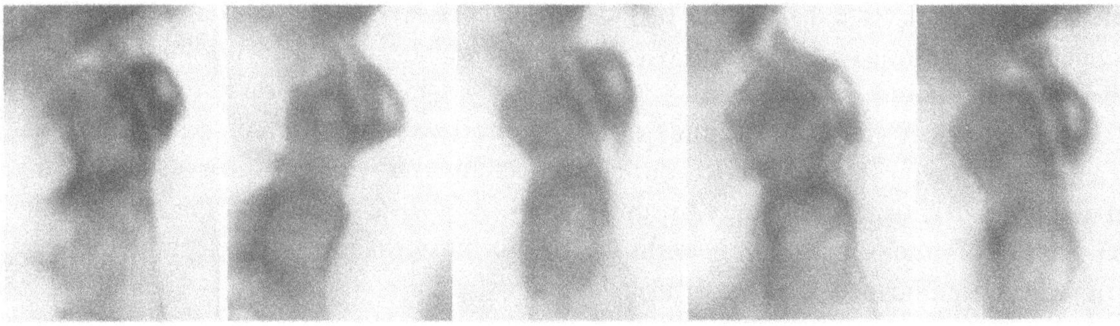

Fig. 31. Hyperostosis seen in lateral views in rheumatoid arthritis

A. Morphology

We classify hyperostoses according to site, extension, and radiographic features in different projections. Indeed, despite their different morphology, these ossifications have similar interpretations.

We should like to emphasize that the diversity in morphology might be partly due to radiographic projection. Thus, rotation or flexion of the head could show the ossification to be attached or continuous with the bones in the cervico-occipital joint, or, conversely, to be a free ossification (Fig. 26).

The adopted classification is as follows:

1. Frontal projections (Fig. 27)
   a. Free ossicle (crowned odontoid)
   b. Ossification of the odontoid
      Apical (median, lateral or total)
      Lateral
   c. Ossification of the atlas
      Superointernal angle
      Internal lateral margin
   d. Combination of these different types
2. Lateral projections (Fig. 28)
   a. Ossification of the clivus
      Free
      Attached to the tip
   b. Ossifications of the odontoid Tip
      Anterior aspect
      Anteroinferior angle
   c. Ossifications of the atlas
      Superior aspect } free or attached
      Inferior aspect } free or attached
   d. Combinations of these different types.

Among the *ossifications visible on frontal views* we describe the "crowned odontoid process" (Figs. 29, 30). This condition is visualized on tomograms and is characterized by the presence of one or several periapical ossicles of extremely variable size, feeble density, and rather irregular edges—sometimes blurred. In its classical form, an ossicle is not continuous with the opacity of the dens. In this case, a lateral view of the ossicle shows it to arise from the upper aspect of the anterior arch of the atlas. In other cases, it is continuous, or at least partly continuous, with the opacity of the odontoid process and with the subapical crown. These cases are consistent with an ossicle which is inserted directly on the apex of the dens. Median as well as latero-apical ossifications provide a "horned aspect" to the apex of the odontoid process, whereas the coating of the entire tip by a bony mass produces a "cauliflower" aspect. When the lateral aspects of the dens are covered with a layer of bone (Figs. 30, 67) its diameter is markedly increased and the lateral atlanto-odontoid space may be almost entirely filled up. This picture is to be distinguished from acquired transverse dislocation of the cervical hinge. For current practice, Wackenheim's rules should be retained:

If asymmetrical spaces are found in a patient without symptoms of cervico-occipital disease, the deformity is due to a simple asymmetry of the bones, i.e. without pathological significance, whereas, if asymmetry is present in a patient with clinical features of cervico-occipital localization, the dislocation is considered pathological. Asymmetry of the lateral atlanto-odontoid interspace may be due to developmental asymmetry of the condyles, the atlas, the axis, or to an acquired asymmetry.

When ossifications of the atlas cover entirely its internal aspect (Fig. 30), they may also narrow this space, but they are more often located in the supero-internal angle of the lateral mass. Finally, we would like to emphasize that we never found ossifications on the occipital condyles.

Also, on *lateral views* a great variety of images are seen (Fig. 31). The inferior extremity of the basilar process, which forms the anterior edge of the foramen magnum, may be deformed by a piriform ossification, which lengthens the clivus. The length of the normal adult clivus is 3.2 ± 0.3 cm (Schmidt and Fischer [311]). Sometimes this opacity is distinct from the basion and merely fills the space between the basion and the tip of the dens. These pictures are usually considered to be consistent with condylus tertius or surnumerary vertebrae.

We have never encountered abnormal growth in the area of the pharyngeal tubercle.

Ossifications of the anterior aspect of the odontoid are located at the level of the anterior tubercle forming there a kind of console on which the anterior arch of the atlas seems to rest. Moreover, there may also exist ossifications of the anteroinferior angle, which resemble syndesmophytes.

On lateral views or on midsagittal tomograms, the anterior arch of the atlas appears normally as a hemispherical structure.

Ossifications occur at the posteroinferior or posterosuperior angle, and are occasionally quite widespread—seeming to articulate at once with the clivus and with the tip of the odontoid process.

B. Signification of Ossifications

Kalenscher's term "accessory eminences" is consistent with bone growth around the foramen magnum due to ossification of the ligamental attachments. Besides, there exists a median and vertical occipitodental ligament stretching from the exocranial aspect of the median part of the anterior edge of the foramen magnum to the tip or sometimes slightly posterior to the tip of the dens. A cartilaginous nodule has been reported to occupy the center of this ligament: it is a vestige of the primitive chord which may also ossify.

Manifestations of the occipital vertebra are also a well-known feature in humans [51, 215, 311, 361, 380, 394]. This area does not exist in fish, but appears in amphibians. Each primary somite has on its internal aspect a mesenchymal condensation which is highly osteogenic: the sclerotome.

Each vertebra is formed from parts of two adjacent sclerotomes. The rearrangement of segmentation results in an alteration in the position of the vertebrae with respect to the myotomes. Thus, the atlas is formed by the caudal part of the first sclerotome and the cranial part of the second sclerotome. A half-sclerotome remains cranial to the first vertebra, i.e. the proatlas. Occasionally, elements of the proatlas may be seen in mammals. They are of two kinds and belong either to perichordal or to hypochordal elements. Concerning the first, the formation of a proatlantal neural arch, or a part thereof, is noted in the Dachs rabbit with chondrodystrophy. As concerns the second ones, a condylus tertius or an isolated ossiculum in front of the foramen magnum may be considered as the hypocentrum or intercentrum of the proatlas.

In a former study [384], on cervical forms of vertebral hyperostosis, we reported on the possible correlations of these ossifications with the osteogenic potential of the prevertebral mesenchyma corresponding to the hemal arch in vertebrates. This arch still exists in dolphins and has totally disappeared in humans. Could hyperostosis of the cervico-occipital joint be viewed as being due to osteogenic potential, i.e. the human remnant of the hemal arch?

All the features we have recorded cannot be correlated with the manifestations of the occipital vertebra. But it is certain that there exists in the cervico-occipital area a cellular material which could be a phylogenic remnant of a feature normally present in fossils and in some groups of vertebrates, or an ontogenic remnant, i.e. virtually present in the embryo but developing accidentally.

The high incidence of such manifestations in ankylosing vertebral hyperostosis, in rheumatoid arthritis, and in psoriasis (cf. Part 6, Chapter 3), leads one to believe that multiple factors could cause this ossification, i.e. traumatic, mechanic, metabolic, inflammatory, etc. For the sake of simplicity we have termed these ossifications *hyperostosis of the cervico-occipital joint.*

Ossification of the ligaments and of the meninges will be dealt with in detail in Part 6, Chapter 2.

Chapter 5 Subluxations-Ligamentous Lesions

Since they have from a clinical and radiological point of view the most striking repercussions, subluxations are the best-known and the most-studied lesions in rheumatoid arthritis. Among them the anterior atlantoaxial subluxation is the most obvious. Nevertheless, other types of subluxations are encountered:

Transverse atlantoaxial subluxation
Atlantoaxial rotation and subluxation
Upward atlantoaxial subluxation
Backward subluxation of the atlas
Forward atlantooccipital subluxation.

These different types are illustrated in Figure 32.

I. Transverse Subluxation [380]

A. Radiographic Technique

Only a tomogram taken in the position with the forehead and nose on the table or an equivalent position can be used for satisfactory detection of transverse subluxations. Only these give a symmetrical radiographic picture of the skull, which allows the different landmarks to be used. The occipital, atlantal and dental anatomic landmarks are subject to variations too wide to be useful for the determination of the midline. The utriculosaccular structure is chosen as a reference because it has, besides its anatomicophysiological value, the advantage of being small and individualized enough for the presence of its right and left pictures on a same section to be a criterion of symmetry of the skull. In practice, a line joining both vestibular shadows of the inner ear is drawn. Then, a perpendicular, representing the intervestibular line, is dropped from the midpoint of this line. Normally, this line passes through the vertical axis of the odontoid process and through the tip of Schmidt and Fischer's condylar angle. The axis of the odontoid may also be added to objectify the midline of the first two vertebrae. In normal cases, these three landmarks coincide and their superposition is a criterion of symmetry of the bones in the craniocervical region. In cases with rheumatoid arthritis, deviations with regard to these axes are consistent with craniocervical asymmetries termed by us transverse subluxations.

B. The Different Types of Transverse Subluxation

Theoretically, three types of subluxations may be distinguished:

Type 1: The interdependent skull-atlas is displaced with regard to the axis of the odontoid. In other words, the intervestibular axis coincides with the bisectrix of the condylar angle, but the two do not coincide

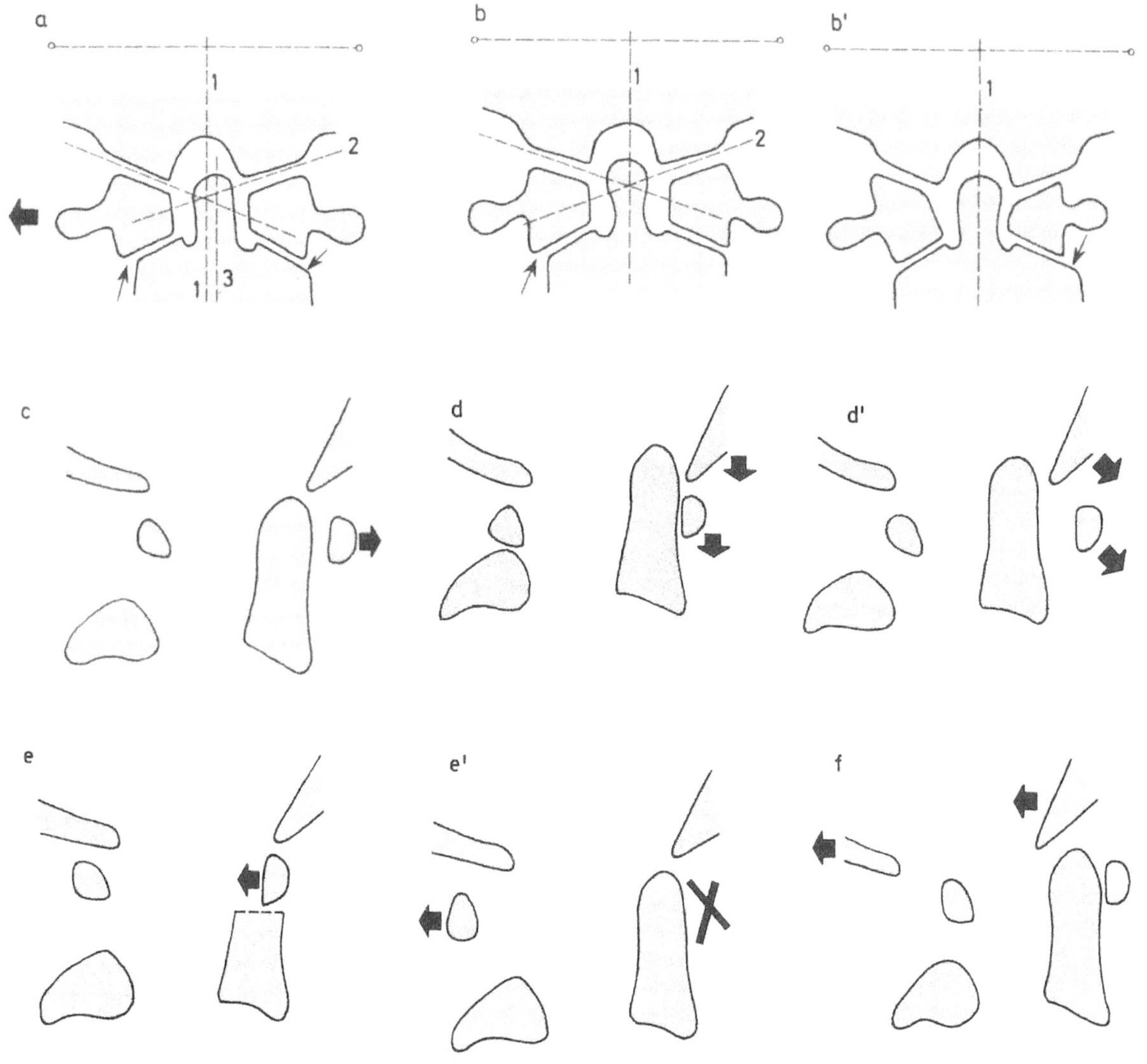

Fig. 32a–f. Subluxations occuring in rheumatoid arthritis. **(a)** Transverse atlantoaxial subluxation. *1* Intervestibular line, *2* Condylar angle, *3* Midline of axis vertebra. **(b)** Rotation subluxation of axis vertebra. **(b′)** Rotation subluxation of atlas. **(c)** Anterior atlantoaxial subluxation. **(d)** Upward atlantoaxial subluxation – in fact inferior or caudal atlantoaxial subluxation. **(d′)** Upward atlantoaxial subluxation with anterior atlantoaxial subluxation. **(e)** Backward subluxation of atlas with lesions of odontoid **(e)** or of anterior arch of the atlas **(e′)**. **(f)** Backward subluxation of occiput

with the axis of the odontoid process. Most often it is a matter of subluxation.

Type 2: The intervestibular axes and the tip of the condylar angle do not coincide. The axis of the odontoid process falls in with one or the other of these cranial axes.

Type 3: The three landmarks do not coincide at all and there is complete transverse subluxation.

The case most often encountered in rheumatic pathology is the transverse atlantoaxial subluxation (Figs. 8, 33). The intervestibular line passes through the tip of the condylar angle, but the axis of the odontoid process is laterally displaced. On one side, the lateral margin of the axis vertebra overlaps that of the atlas and on the other side, it is the margin of the atlas that overlaps the axis. Finally, the lateral atlantodental

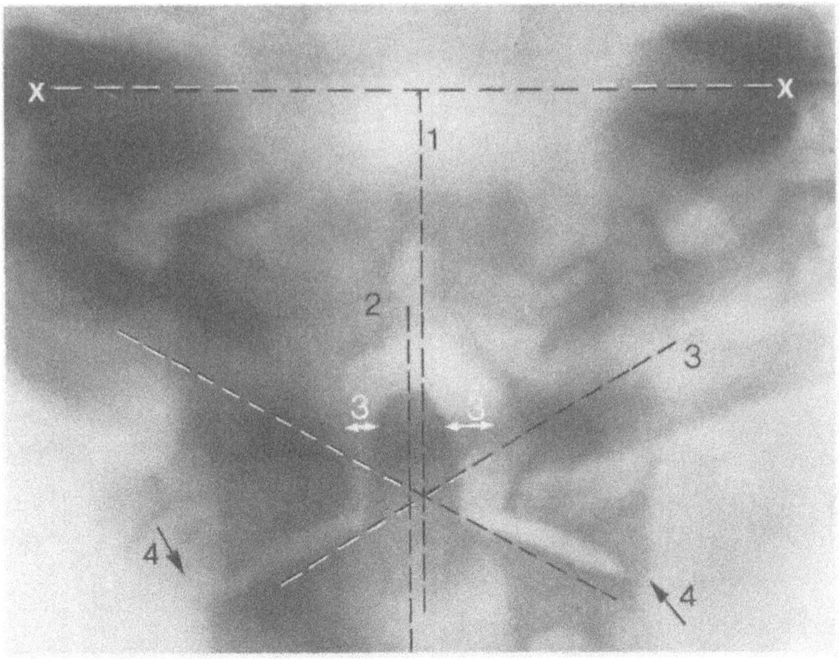

Fig. 33. Transverse subluxation of atlas toward the left in rheumatoid arthritis. Intervestibular line *(1)* is shifted laterally with respect to the midline of the dens *(2)*. The condylar angle *(3)* coincides with the intervestibular line. Asymmetrical spaces between the lateral aspect of the odontoid and the lateral masses of the atlas *(4)*. Disalignment of the left and right side at the level of the atlantoaxial interspace

interspace is wider on one side. It should be noted that transverse subluxation is often associated with rotation subluxation.

C. Provoked Transverse Subluxation

As anterior atlantoaxial subluxation may be revealed by a functional study, i.e. by flexion movement, so evidence of transverse subluxation may be provided by lateroflexion (Fig. 34). Thinking that this examination would provide useful data concerning articular and ligamental laxity, we carried it out in more than 80 cases. However, from a technical point of view, this has not always been easy, and in more than half of the cases associated rotation could not be avoided, rendering the X-ray uninterpretable for lateral flexion. In the other cases, rational interpretation has not been possible. Some patients with lesions of the transverse ligament, i.e. anterior atlantoaxial subluxation, had also a provoked transverse subluxation on one or on both sides. Contrariwise, other cases showed no transverse subluxation. Finally, some patients without anterior subluxation had transverse subluxation on one side or on both.

To conclude, it may be said that it has not been possible to draw definite conclusions. This examination has been rather disappointing. In patients where it had been possible to perform this examination several times, sometimes after 3 years, the findings varied greatly, e.g., induced transverse subluxations became spontaneous subluxations and, inversely, patients with induced subluxations did not present signs of transverse subluxation at subsequent examinations.

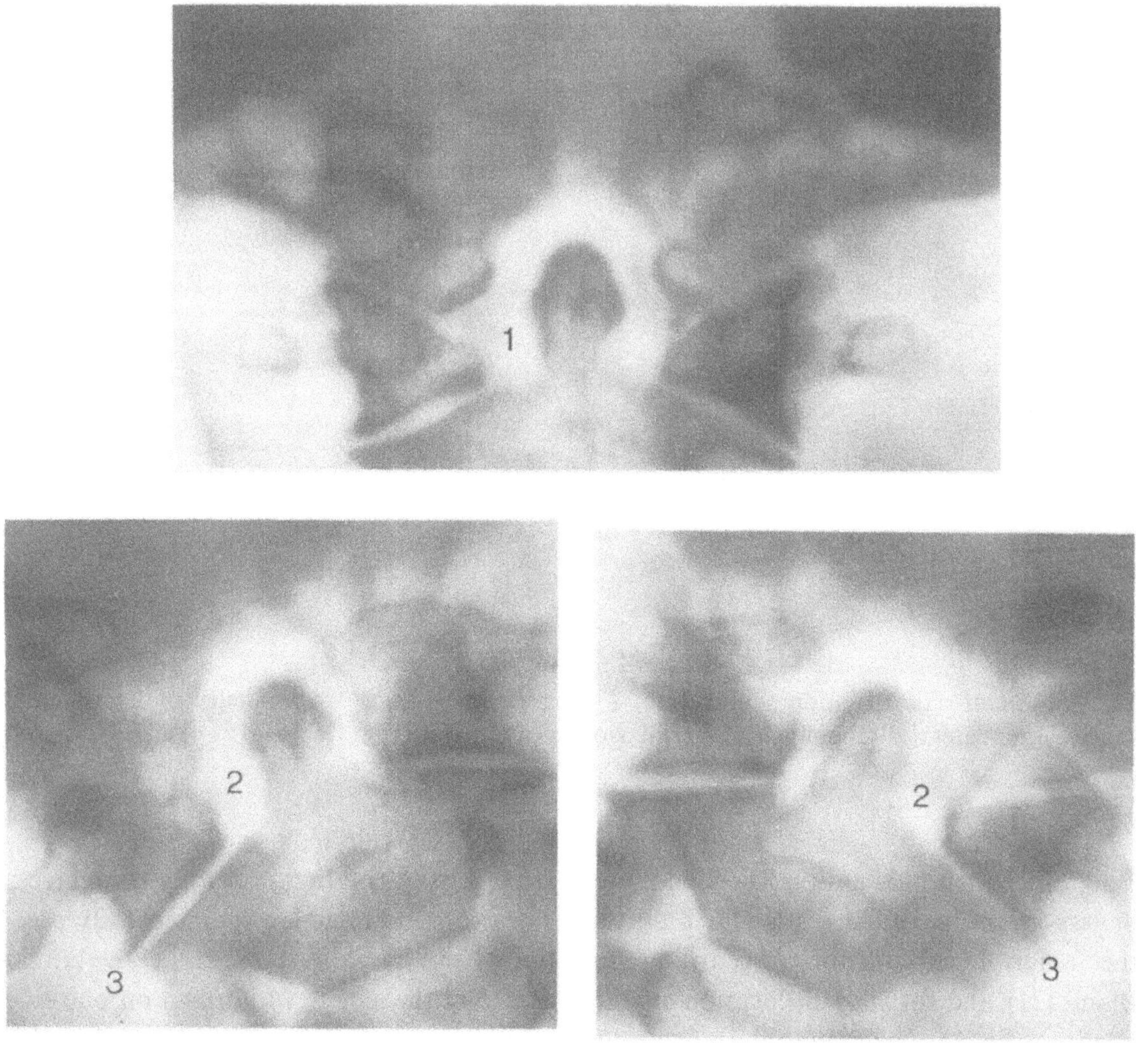

Fig. 34. Lateroflexion aimed at demonstrating instability of a lateral atlantoaxial subluxation. The laterodental interspace is symmetrical in the neutral position *(1)*, and changes its width in left and right lateral flexion *(2)*. The lateral disalignment changes according to the side of the lateral flexion *(3)*

D. Irreducible Transverse Subluxation

Transverse subluxations may be reduced by lateroflexion. However, when there is a significant destruction of the articular interspaces between the lateral masses of atlas and axis, lateroflexion no longer reduces the subluxation because ankylosis has occurred and the bone fragments are interlocked (Fig. 49).

II. Subluxation and Rotation

[27, 36, 173, 221, 344, 380, 396]

It seems that rotation has been partly overlooked in connection with subluxations of the craniocervical joint in chronic inflammatory rheumatism. The first studies on atlantoaxial subluxations all mentioned the rotatory component (Malgaigne [221]; Berkheiser and Seidler [27]; Hess et al. [173]; Sullivan [344]; Boever and Hennebert

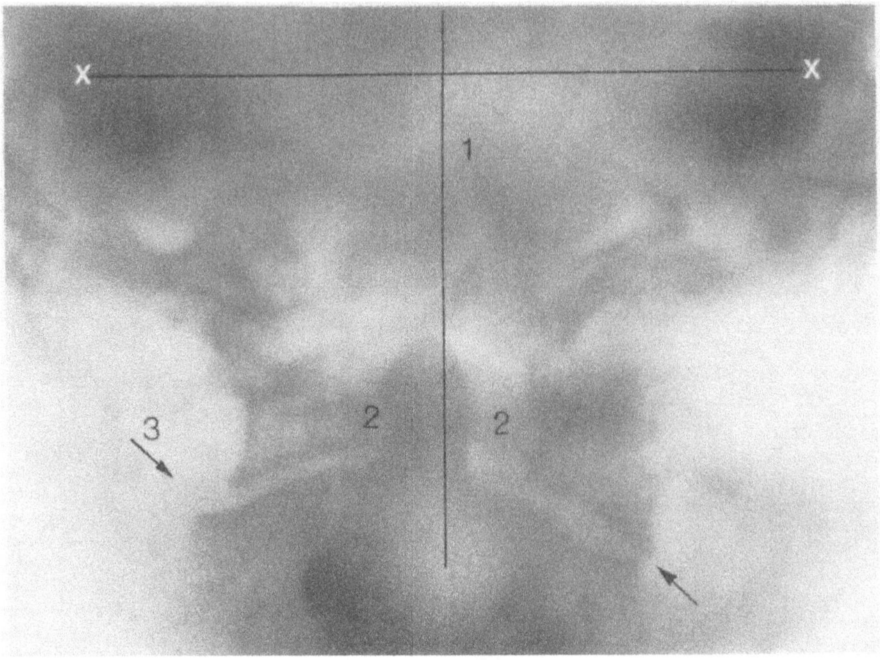

Fig. 35. Atlantoaxial rotation subluxation. *1* Intervestibular line, *2* Asymmetry of laterodental spaces, *3* Unilateral disalignment of lateral aspects of C1 and C2 vertebrae

[36]). Since then, this notion has been more or less given up and stress is laid only on the anterior subluxation. According to Bland [31], the forward dislocation of the atlas may be more pronounced on one side, and we have the same opinion (Fig. 39). Others, e.g., Martel [225], consider this interpretation improbable because stretching of the transverse ligament must result in equal displacement of both sides of the lateral atlantoaxial joint, which possesses lax joint capsules. Werne [396], however, gave a detailed description of different types of anterior atlantoaxial subluxation combined with rotation, and he distinguished the following:

Unilateral dislocation backward
Unilateral dislocation forward
Bilateral dislocation forward with or without rotation
Unilateral dislocation forward with controlateral dislocation backward.

Atlantoaxial rotation is readily recognized. The skull and atlas are symmetrically positioned and the axis is rotated, i.e. the lateral aspect of the axis is withdrawn on one side with respect to the lateral mass of the atlas (Figs. 9, 32b, 35). The axis is in the symmetrical position, and the skull and the atlas are rotated, i.e., the lateral aspect of the lateral mass of the atlas is withdrawn on one side with respect to the axis (Fig. 32b′).

III. Anterior Atlantoaxial Subluxation

This is the most commonly encountered and also the best known lesion of the craniocervical joint in rheumatoid arthritis. It consists in forward displacement of the atlas-skull and is usually referred to as atlantoaxial subluxation (let us also recall that subluxation and diastasis may be used as synonyms). To give evidence of a widening of the atlantoaxial interspace, which is the main criterion of subluxation, the radiological examination of the upper cervical spine must comprise, besides the statics, a functional study. Indeed, quite a number of subluxations are only recognized in the flexion position.

A. Radiological Technique

As we already pointed out, our routine roentgenologic examination comprises:

1. A strictly lateral plain film of the cervical spine with the patient in the sitting position. Care must be taken that the head is in the ortho-optic position with the hard palate horizontal. This is achieved by placing the lower rim of the orbits on the same horizontal plane as the external auditory meatus.

2. A lateral projection in the flexion position with the patient tucking the chin in. We already spoke about the importance of this position, but we would like to stress it once more since the correct interpretation of the functional study depends on it. Indeed, it is compulsory to have only one type of movement.

3. A lateral projection taken in the hyperextension position. There too, the correct extension of the upper cervical region is obtained by drawing the head forward as far as possible and then extending it, without moving the neck backward.

These three projections may also be used in tomography since median or paramedian tomograms provide more information and allow more precise measurements with a constant magnification coefficient.

B. Normal Values of the Anterior Atlantodental Articular Interspace

Normally, there is no diastasis at this level, and the width of the interspace should not exceed 2.5 mm in flexion. Coutts [81] found it to have a mean value of 2 mm and Jackson a maximal value of 2.5 mm in adults and 3 mm in children [184]. Serre et al. [316] carried out a study on 84 cases without inflammatory diseases and demonstrated that the atlantoodontoid interspace is normally, in children, 2 mm or more in the neutral position, and up to 4 mm in the flexion position, whereas above the age of 20 it measures between 1.0 and 1.8 mm in the neutral position and 1.5 to 2.4 in the flexion position. The distance is measured at the level of the middle part of the anterior arch of the atlas.

We consider pathological spaces measuring at least –

2.5 mm in adults in the neutral position or in flexion;

3.0 mm in children in the neutral position; and

4.5 mm in children in flexion.

C. Measurements of Atlantoaxial Subluxation

Though widening of the atlantoaxial interspace is the sign that draws attention, it is only an indirect sign. The measurement of the atlantoaxial diastasis is usually made from the middle of the posterior aspect of the anterior arch of the atlas to the anterior edge of the odontoid process. We have been using the same technique so as to permit comparison of the results with those of other authors. In fact, the margins of this

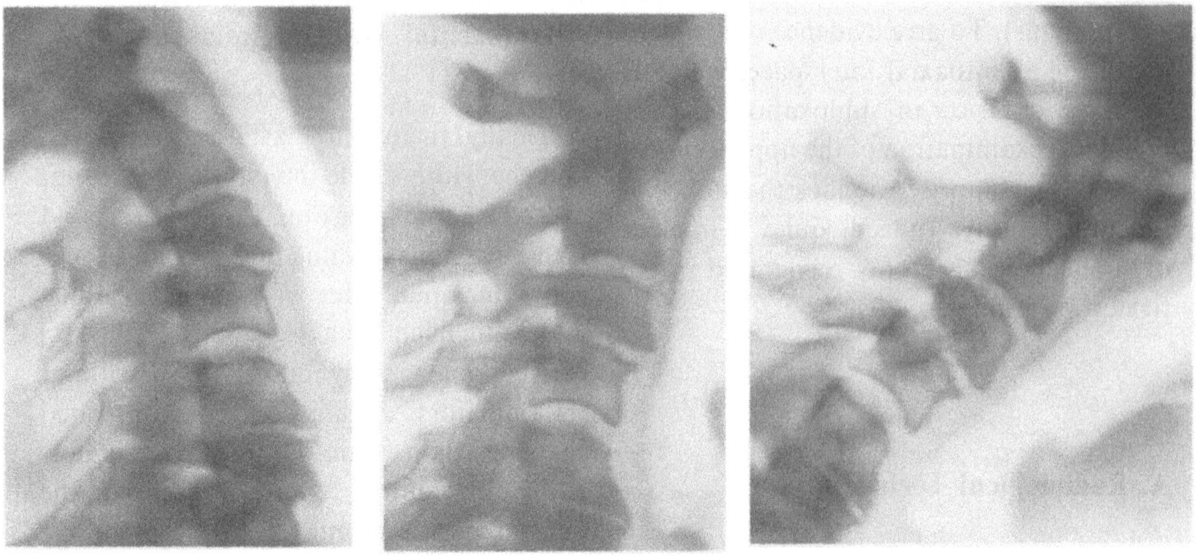

Fig. 36. Important and classical anterior atlantoaxial subluxation, still reducible in extension (a). Note multiple fixed spondylodiscitis in C3/4, C5/6 and C6/7, with anterior subluxation of C3 on C4 and C6 on C7

interspace may not be parallel, due to some deflection of the atlas. The measurement of the longest distance between the anterior arch of the atlas and the odontoid process would provide a better account of the spinal cord involvement.

As a matter of fact, the measurement of the diastasis is convenient and easy, but does not give exact information about the narrowing of the spinal canal, i.e. the pathogenic lesion.

The measurement of displacement of the odontoid process behind the basilar line is no more precise. Theoretically, the displacement would be equal to the diastasis but under two conditions, first, that origi-

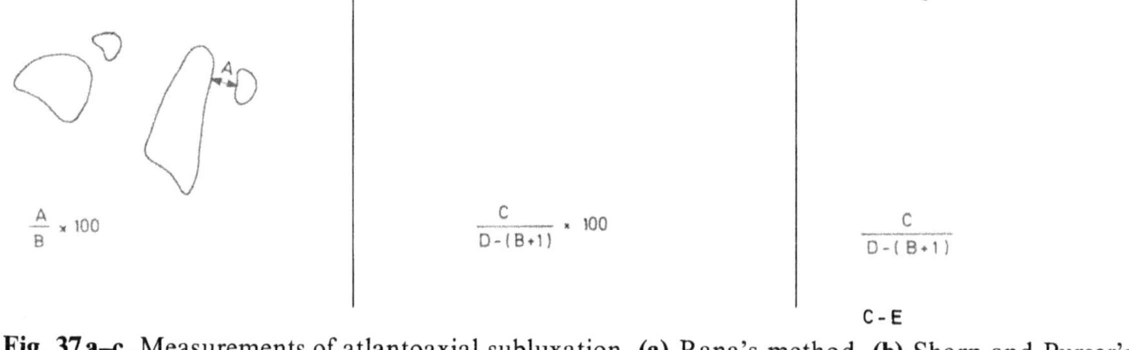

Fig. 37 a–c. Measurements of atlantoaxial subluxation. **(a)** Rana's method. **(b)** Sharp and Purser's method. **(c)** Author's method

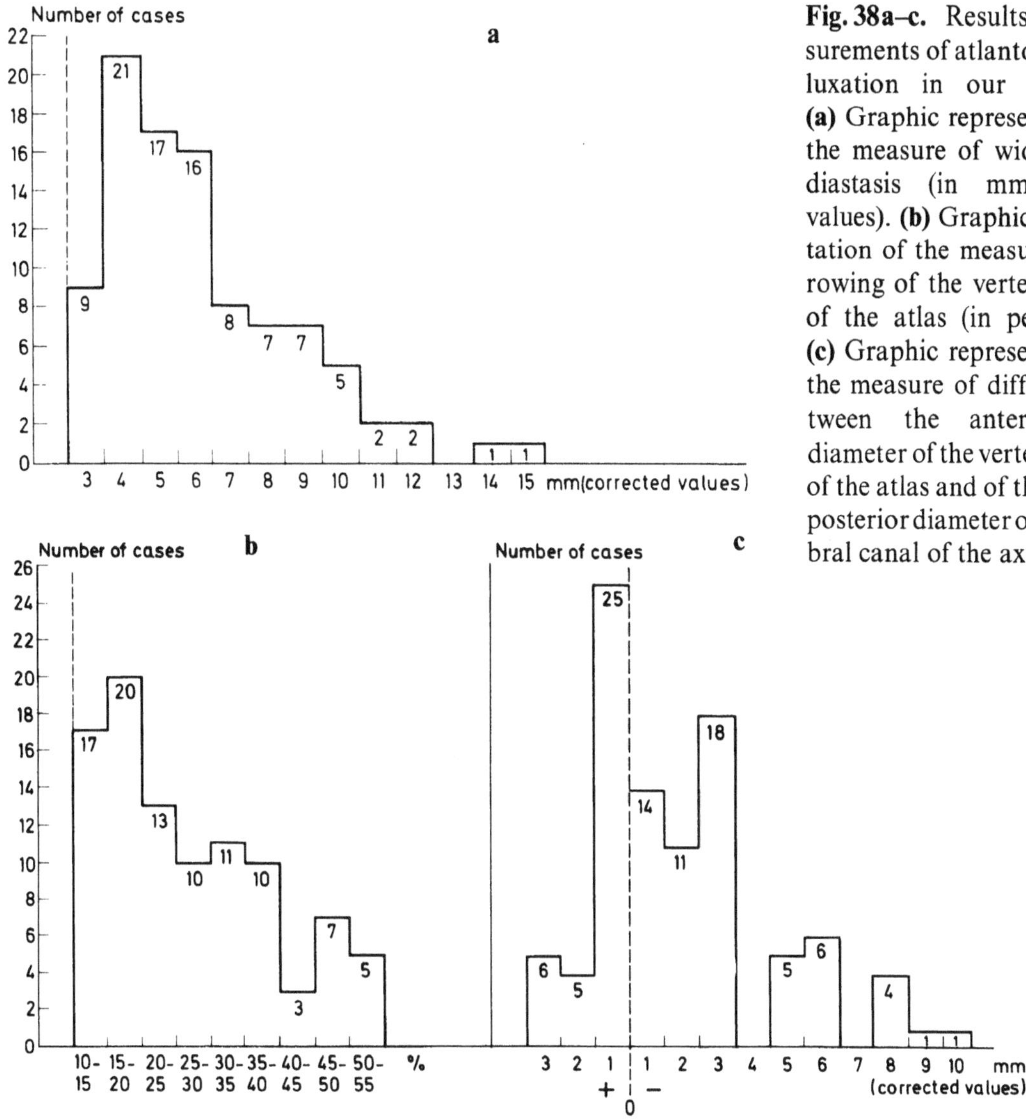

Fig. 38a–c. Results of measurements of atlantoaxial subluxation in our 96 cases. **(a)** Graphic representation of the measure of width of the diastasis (in mm-corrected values). **(b)** Graphic representation of the measure of narrowing of the vertebral canal of the atlas (in percentage). **(c)** Graphic representation of the measure of difference between the anteroposterior diameter of the vertebral canal of the atlas and of the anterioposterior diameter of the vertebral canal of the axis (in mm)

nally the odontoid process be tangent to the basilar line, and second, that no upward luxation exist besides the anterior subluxation.

The main measurement is that of the narrowing of the spinal canal.

To appreciate the percentage narrowing of the spinal canal, Rana et al. [282] (Fig. 37a) effected two measurements: (1) the distance *a* separating the anterior surface of the dens from the posterior aspect of the anterior arch of the atlas in flexion, and, (2) the distance *b* separating the posterior surface of the dens from the anterior surface of the posterior arch in extension. The percentage narrowing of the spinal canal could thus be calculated as $(a/b) \times 100$. This measure is valuable only when the atlantoaxial subluxation is entirely reducible.

According to Sharp and Purser [324] (Fig. 37b) the anteroposterior diameter of the spinal canal on the film taken in flexion was measured as the shortest distance between the anterior surface of the posterior arch of the atlas and the posterior surface of the odontoid process. This was expressed as a percentage to the nearest 5%. The original size of the spinal canal was estimated by subtracting the anteroposterior diameter

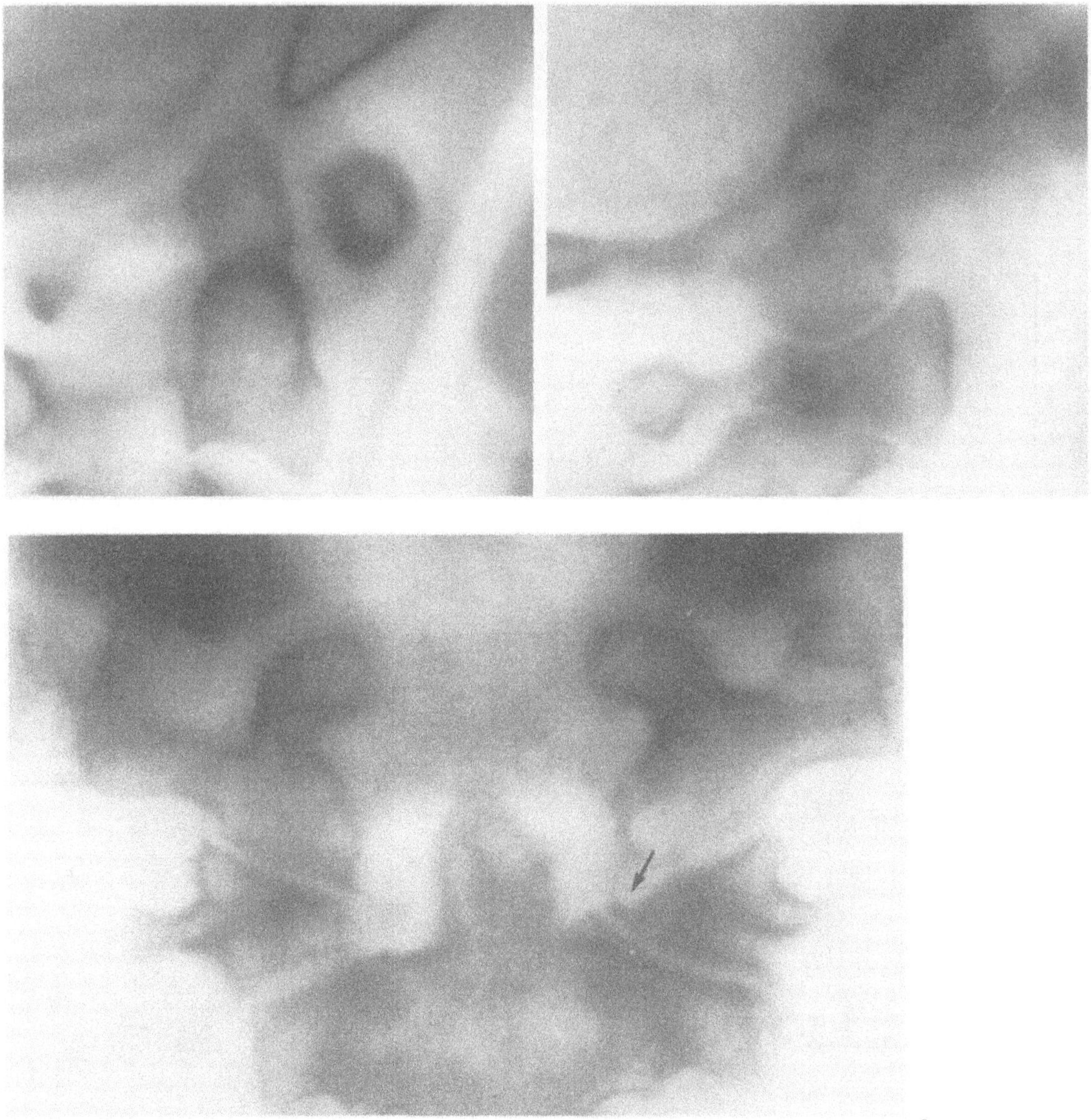

a b c

Fig. 39a–c. Association of four subluxations in a case of juvenile chronic polyarthritis in a 20-year-old patient. **(a)** Anterior atlantoaxial and moderate upward odontoid subluxations. Note hypertrophic anterior arch of atlas, which may be correlated with early onset of the disease. **(b)** Anterior atlantoaxial subluxation. Note normal shape and size of the posterior arch in this lateral tomographic section with respect to its image in the median section **(a)**. This is due to the rotation subluxation **(c)**. **(c)** Rotation atlantoaxial subluxation. Note presence of osteophytes in this young patient

of the odontoid process, plus an arbitrary 1 mm for the original depth of the atlantoaxial joint, from the distance between the anterior surface of the posterior arch and the posterior surface of the anterior arch of the atlas. The calculation is represented by the formula:

$$\frac{C}{D-(B+1)} \times 100.$$

In addition, these authors demonstrate that the reduction of the spinal canal of the atlas is not only due to the diastasis but depends partly on the inclination of the atlas on the axis. Indeed, the main determinant of the degree of narrowing of the spinal canal was the increase in depth of the anterior atlantoaxial joint, but extreme degrees of inclination further increase the narrowing of the canal (Fig. 53).

As concerns our measurements, and in order to express better the narrowing of the spinal canal of the atlas, we gave the percentage not as the remaining percentage but as the narrowing percentage of the canal. Thus, when the canal measures 85% of its primary diameter, the reduction of the diameter will be 15%.

We also measured the anteroposterior diameter of the spinal canal at the level of the axis and compared it with the anteroposterior diameter of the spinal canal at the level of the atlas. We believe the risk of cord compression to be prominent when the diameter is narrowed at the level of the atlas (Fig. 37c) Wackenheim [380] pointed out that the anteroposterior diameter of the atlas is larger than the anteroposterior diameter of the axis in normal conditions. The same diameter in both vertebrae is the first degree of narrowing. But when the anteroposterior diameter of the atlas is smaller, the condition is considered pathological.

More precise data allowing at once measurement of the diameter of the spinal canal and the thickness of the soft tissues would be provided by tomographic gas myelography performed in various head positions.

D. Results of Our Study

Among our 207 examinations carried out on 174 patients with rheumatoid arthritis, we found 96 atlantoaxial subluxations. In fact, some of the patients with atlantoaxial subluxations were X-rayed several times and there were actually only 78 patients with subluxations. But measurements were taken on 96 X-rays, a certain number of subluxations having developed.

1. Spontaneous and Provoked Diastasis; Reducible and Irreducible Diastasis

Among the 96 cases with diastasis, 29 are spontaneous (Fig. 17) and 67 appear at flexion. These are classical data. Sometimes spontaneous subluxation may be aggravated by the flexion movement. We found eight cases in which flexion increases the diastasis. But among the 29 cases of spontaneous subluxation, 12 are reduced by the extension movement (Fig. 36). Finally, only 17 are irreducible. No previous publications reported reducibility by extension, but on account of our experience, we would advise that the extension movement always be performed in order to prove the irreducibility.

2. What are the Causes of Irreducibility of the Diastasis by the Extension Movement?

The study of our 17 cases showed in each case marked destruction of one or both atlantoaxial joints. Sometimes there exists even fusion or ankylosis between the lateral masses of the atlas and the superior articular facets of the axis. All these cases had quite advanced rheumatoid arthritis. Another hypothesis concerning the irreducibility is given by Kao et al. [190], who postulate that the failure to reduce the dislocation might be explained by the presence of rheumatoid granulation tissue between the anterior arch of C1 vertebra and the odontoid process. This presence of rheumatoid granulation tissue is mentioned in some post-mortem reports [31, 118, 190, 230].

3. Importance of the Diastasis: Minor, Definite, Major

Along with other authors [69, 316, 324], we adopted the following classification to characterize the degree of atlantoaxial subluxation:

Minor diastasis: less than 5 mm	47 cases
Definite diastasis: 5–8 mm	31 cases
Major diastasis: more than 9 mm	18 cases

The importance of the diastasis is not always consistent with the degree of narrowing of the atlantal canal. In our material, we only consider the anteroposterior diameter to characterize the size of the bony canal proper. Sharp and Purser demonstrated the narrowing to be mainly determined by the increased atlantoaxial interval, extreme degrees of inclination of the atlas, either forward or backward, further increasing the narrowing of the canal. Besides, and taking into account that the odontoid process commonly broadens out inferiorly, associated upward subluxation also increases the narrowing. In such cases, however, there is often erosion of the odontoid as well as of its posterior and its apical aspects. The narrowing of the canal will then be less marked.

This is the reason why we measured the degree of narrowing of the canal and expressed it by percentage. Figure 38b displays our data.

In 71 cases the narrowing of the atlantal canal is less than 30%, in 20 cases it is 30–50% and in five cases, more than 50%.

Finally, we compared the anteroposterior diameter of the vertebral canal at the level of the atlas with the corresponding anteroposterior diameter at the level of the axis. We have already pointed out that the sagittal diameter at the level of the atlas measures normally 1–3 mm more than at the level of the axis. Figure 38c indicates the difference between those two diameters, and shows that—

in 36 cases the C1 diameter was larger than the C2,

in 59 cases the C1 diameter was smaller than the C2,

in 41 cases smaller by 1–4 mm, and

in 18 cases smaller by 5–10 mm.

All these measurements do not, however, allow precise rules to be drawn concerning atlantoaxial subluxation with neurological complications, but they permit a better approach to the problem. Moreover, it is very likely that other factors play a determining role as concerns the neurological disturbances. A marked subluxation, which has occurred rather progressively and is then fixed, may be better tolerated than a less marked but unstable one in which each flexion-extension movement causes cord compression.

4. Rotation or Translation Associated with Atlantoaxial Subluxation

Werne [396] gave an accurate account of the different mechanisms associating rotation with atlantoaxial subluxation. But though these displacements are not uninteresting, they are most of the time too small to be visible on X-rays, so that only marked rotations are readily diagnosed. We already recorded the radiological characteristics of these rotations, but the measurement of the angle of rotation is almost impossible. We also stated that one can speak of arthritis of the atlantoaxial articulations only if these cannot be visualized on any of the tomographic sections. Rotation by itself, may cause the articular interspace to become invisible on some section planes.

Finally, rotation associated with atlantoaxial subluxation may partly account for the neurological complications being unilateral. As Perovic et al. [271] suppose, the spinal cord could be pushed aside or even twisted to some extent. The roentgen appearance of atlantoaxial subluxation has been dealt with. Such a lesion, sometimes small, is frequently seen to be associated with anterior atlantoaxial subluxation. As with rotation, the displacement is not readily measurable. Finally, anterior atlantoaxial subluxation may be associated at once with rotation subluxation and with transverse subluxation (Fig. 39). This condition comprising several anteroposterior and lateral displacements is characteristic of rheumatic diseases due to the multiple locations of synovial, ligamentous lesions, and also to articular and bone destructions.

E. Radiodynamic Examination in Atlantoaxial Subluxation

1. Author's Method

We carried out the dynamic examination in 96 cases of atlantoaxial subluxation. In 60 cases only plain X-rays were performed, whereas 36 also had tomograms.

a) Radiodynamic Examination of the Cervico-Occipital Region

The physiological movement being known, we describe several pathological functional circumstances (Fig. 40). In the absence of diastasis, the following features are encountered:

Type 1: This consists in accentuation of the physiological rocking motion of the atlas. The movement is functionally harmonious and probably is only due to hyperlaxity of the transverse ligament and cannot be definitely related to the rheumatic disease. There is no associated osteoarticular lesion (Fig. 40,*1*).

Type 2: This is the same movement as type 1 but associated with C0/1 block. (Wackenheim describes a peculiar dynamic feature occurring during the flexion-extension movement; on lateral X-rays, the connections between the occiput and the atlas remain unchanged in the three positions and the atlas moves without changing its connections with the occiput.) Rather than "functional block," we would call it "block of function." Indeed, in some cases, we found evidence of osteoarticular lesions (Fig. 40,*2*)

When there is a subluxation, we distinguish two other types:

Type 3. It consists in an authentic flexion-diastasis of more than 3 mm, reducible by extension.

It is a harmonious movement with gaping and progressive bringing together of the posterior arch of the atlas and the occipital squama. Diastasis occurs during flexion and the vector A-A′ tends to be horizontal as in a shearing movement. The diastasis has parallel margins, the posterior margin of the anterior arch of the atlas being parallel to the anterior margin of the odontoid (Fig. 40,*3a*). The most frequent case is C0/1 block of function associated with diastasis. Then the rocking motion of the atlas is more marked than the anteroposterior shearing movement, and the vector A-A′ has an obliquely descending direction. The diastasis gaps superiorly (Fig. 40,*3b*).

C1/2 block of function associated with the diastasis is more rare. Its consequence seems to be diastasis with parallel margins caused by the horizontal displacement of

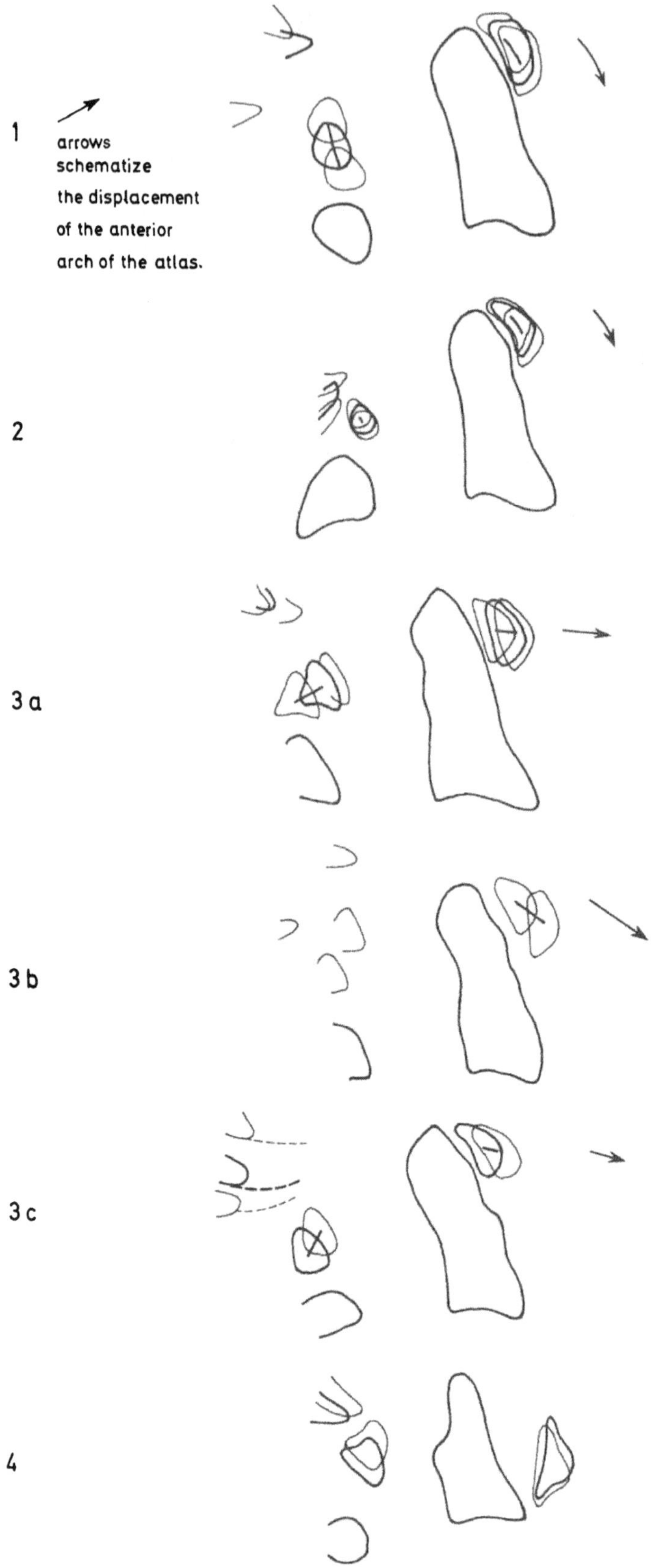

Fig. 40. Radiodynamic study of the cervico-occipital region under pathological circumstances. Author's method (see Part 5, Chapt. 5). **(1)** and **(2)** Polyarthritis without atlantoaxial dislocation. **(3a)** Shearing movement with C0/1 functional block. **(3b)** Shearing movement and gaping. **(3c)** Shearing movement with C1/2 functional block. **(4)** Very reduced mobility in a not-quite-fixed diastasis

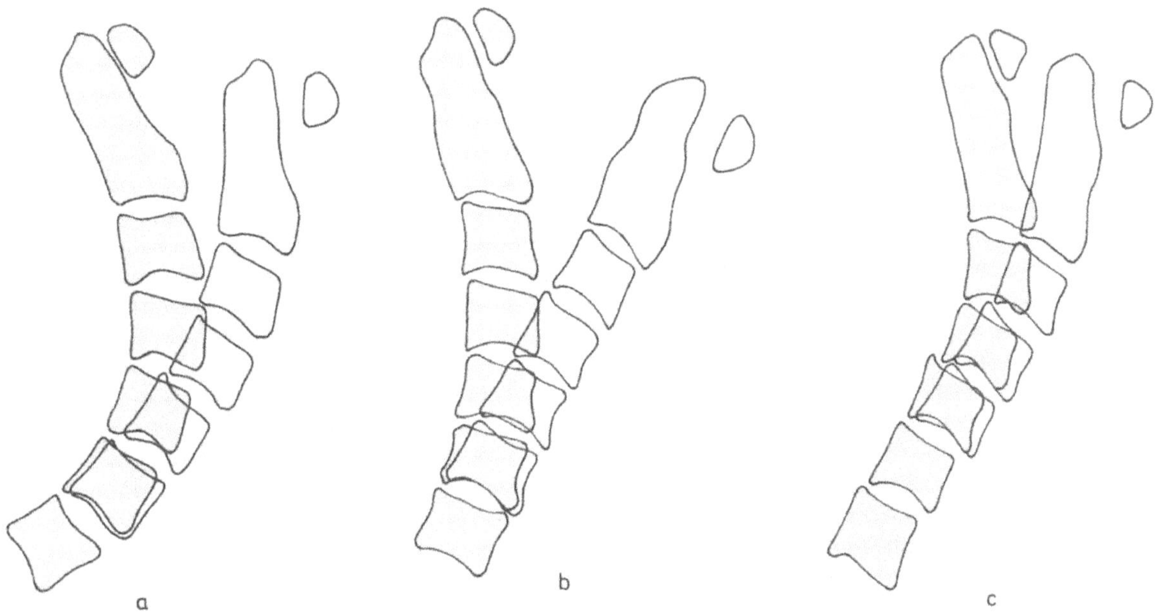

Fig. 41 a–c. Three types of dynamic behavior of the lower cervical spine in atlantoaxial diastasis. **(a)** Fixed lordosis. **(b)** Rectitude in the flexed position. **(c)** Shaped deformation (lordosis of the cervical spine from C1 to C4 and fixed lower cervical spine from C5 to C7)

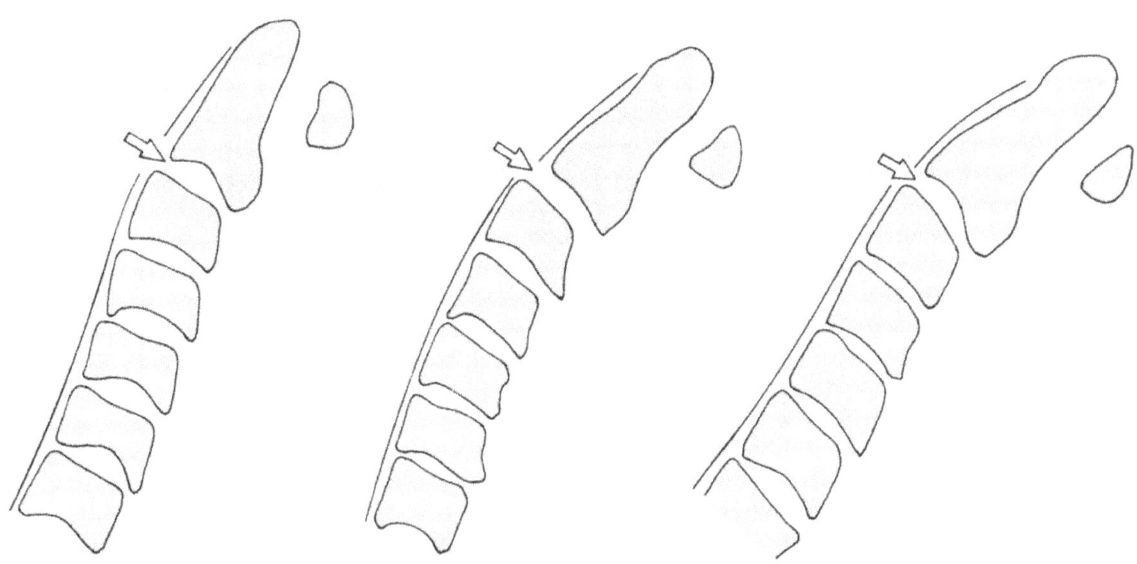

Fig. 42. Drawing of flexed position in three out of nine cases of subluxations of C2/3 vertebrae in rheumatoid arthritis (C2–C3 kyphosis), with irreducible atlantoaxial subluxation

the anterior arch of the atlas and thus of the A-A′ vector (Fig. 40,*3c*).

Type 4. This consists in irreducible diastasis associated with marked destructive osteoarticular lesions, either atlantocondylar or atlantoaxial, or even both. Most of the time, there is also upward subluxation. The posterior movements, between the occipital squama and the posterior arches of atlas and axis are very restricted, mostly insignificant at C0/1 and minimal at C1/2 (Fig. 40,*4*).

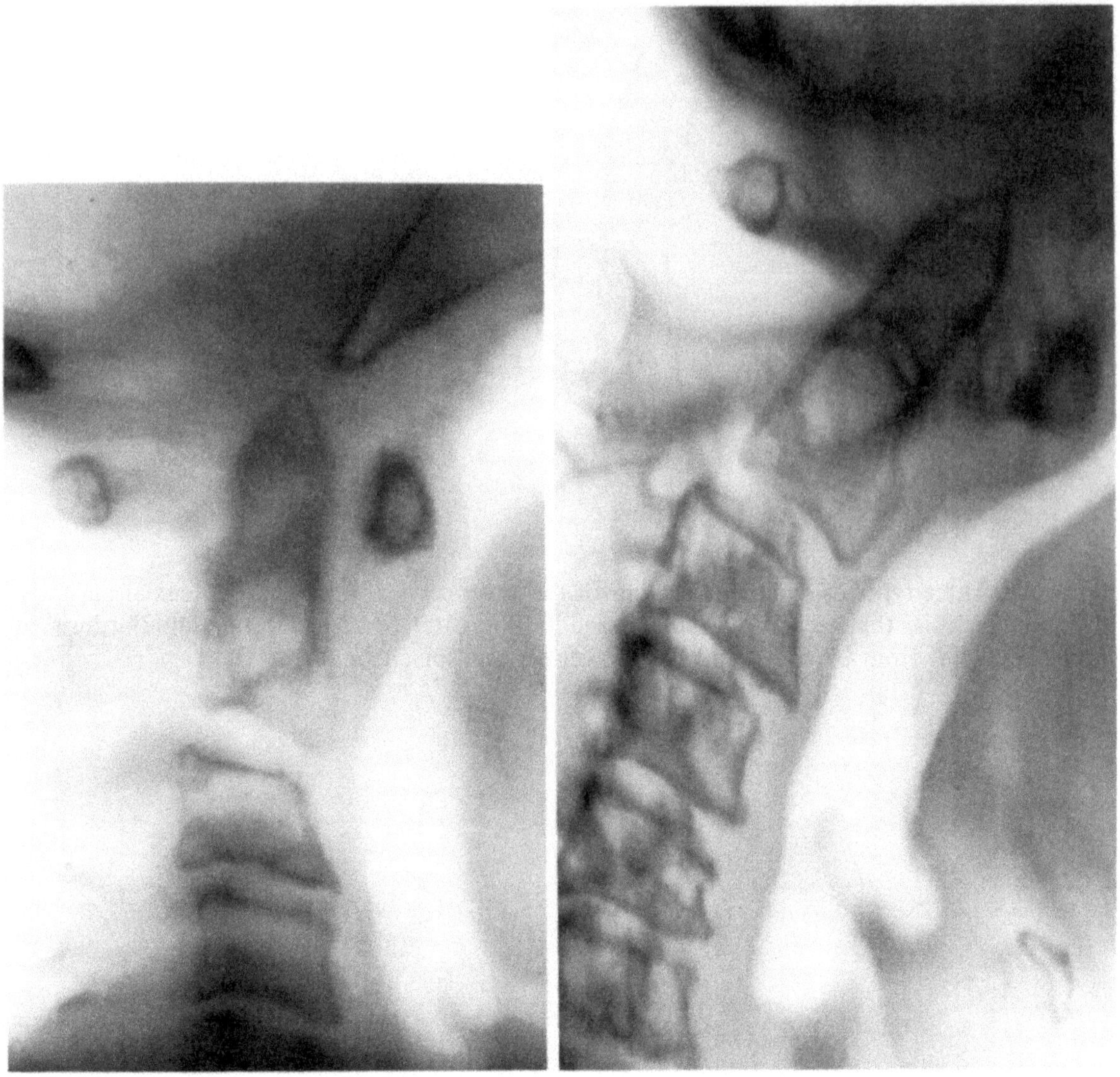

Fig. 43. Compensatory hypermobility and subluxation (kyphosis) in C2/3 connections in two cases of irreducible anterior atlantoaxial subluxation. Three cases out of our nine are schematized in Fig. 42

All these diastases have a common factor, i.e. incompetence or even destruction of the transverse ligament, with perturbations in the cervicocranial dynamics. The occipitoatlantal function would be the first to be reduced because hyperlaxity facilitates the amplitude of the C1/2 flexion. In the C0/1 block-of-function the rocking motion of the atlas predominates. Contrariwise, a shearing movement of the atlas with regard to the axis corresponds to a small gaping of the spinous processes of C1/2.

b) Correlations between the Function Perturbations in the Cervico-Occipital Joint and the Rheumatic Lesions in the C0/1 and C1/2 Articulations

The articulations between occiput. atlas, and axis may be more or less destroyed and it is not always easy to give evidence of minimal degrees of destruction. The articulations move differently owing to the stage of destruction. At the beginning, there is hypermobility, but later on ankylosis occurs due to the complete destruction of the interspaces. A follow-up study would be of interest, but our actual state of research does not allow us to draw absolute rules.

c) Correlations between the Functional Perturbations in the Cervico-Occipital Joint and in the Lower Cervical Spine

The study of the dynamic behavior of the lower cervical spine leads to a description of the four main types of mobility with regard to the functional perturbations observed (Figs. 41, 42).

Normal flexion and extension behavior or only a small restriction in the amplitude of the extension may be observed.

Another type consists in fixed lordosis, which persists in the flexed position of the head (Fig. 41 a). In the third and most frequent type, the range of flexion is limited and there is an overall straightness (Fig. 41 b).

Finally, one may encounter an S-shaped deformation of the spine. One possibility would be the S-shaped deformation – lordosis of the cranial part and kyphosis of the caudal part or vice versa – in the neutral position and accentuated in flexion (Fig. 41 c). In other cases, flexion brings about angular deformation of the spine, the tip of this angle being located at C2/3 when there is an obvious rheumatic involvement of the cervico-occipital joints. In 9 of our 96 cases with atlantoaxial subluxation, the common lesion was C1/2 ankylosis with important and irreducible C1/2 diastasis (Fig. 42). It would seem that C2/3 kyphosis in flexion is the preferential compensation mode in these cases with irreducible diastasis (Fig. 43).

2. Wackenheim's Method [381]

This method consists of taking as a fix the contours of the C7 vertebral body and superimposing on the three fundamental positions. Then, for each of these positions, the posterior aspect of the vertebrae and Chamberlain's line are drawn on the same diagram. This tracing is readily done and provides the diagram depicted in Figure 4. The characteristics of the flexion and extension movements from C2 to C7 are easily recognized and eventually measured. The triangle formed by the Chamberlain lines indicates by its shape as well as by its size the type and the amount of flexion and of extension of the whole cervical spine, the cervico-occipital joint included. Alterations in size and shape of the triangle indicate disturbance in the cervico-occipital function when the mobility between C2 and C7 is normal. Figure 44 depicts the results of this type of study in six cases of rheumatoid arthritis and, thus, demonstrates the method.

3. Penning's Method [270]

This is a simple though somewhat lengthy method for measuring the angular displacement of one vertebra with regard to the other during the flexion-extension movement. Penning reports values of $-6°$ to $30°$ for the C0/1 segment, and of 3 to $35°$ for the C1/2 segment. He points out that "in the total excursion C0/2 the atlanto-occipital segment may play the larger or the smaller part. A mean value for the sagittal movement C0/1 is 25–30°."

In all cases with diastasis, we have found a more or less important reduction in mobility of not only the C0/1, but also, though more moderate, of the C1/2. The mobility of the C2/3 segment is usually 5

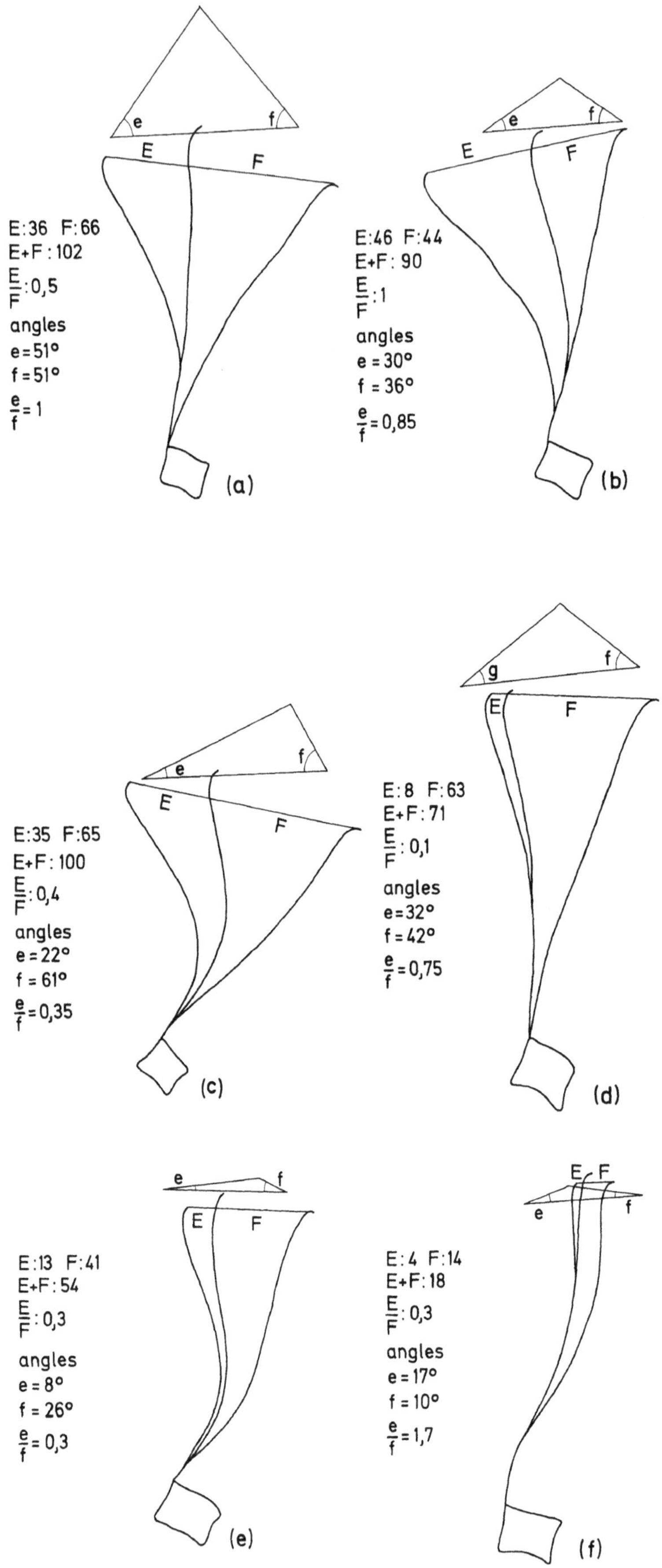

Fig. 44a–f. Wackenheim's method used for study of the mobility of cervico-occipital region and lower cervical spine in six cases of rheumatoid arthritis. **(a)** Moderate reduction of extension movement in the cervical spine ($E/F = 0.5$) compensated by the cervico-occipital hinge ($e/f = 1$). **(b)** Moderate reduction of flexion movement in the cervical spine compensated by the cervico-occipital hinge. **(c)** Non-compensated reduction of extension movement. **(d)** Well compensated reduction of extension movement ($E/F = 0.1$) ($e/f = 0.75$). **(e)** Noncompensated diffuse reduction of the mobility. **(f)** Stiffness of the whole cervical spine. Note overlapping of Chamberlain's line (upward atlantoaxial subluxation)

to 16°. According to Penning, this rather reduced mobility—with regard to the subjacent segments—may be explained by the relative large size of the spinous process of the axis.

In our cases with angular kyphosis, we measured a mean value of 18.5° at the level of C2/3, i.e. a similar value to what Penning records at C3/4, C4/5 and C5/6. This is an example of the utilization of Penning's method to demonstrate hypermobility between two vertebrae.

F. Frequency of Atlantoaxial Subluxation

In 1961 Sharp and Purser [324] carried out a study on 79 in-patients with rheumatoid arthritis, 74 of whom had had a complete roentgen examination. They counted 14 atlantoaxial subluxations, i.e. 18.9% of the X-rayed group. Besides, these authors studied 1,478 subjects taken at random among the population of Leigh to establish the incidence of rheumatoid arthritis. X-rays of the cervical spine in the neutral position revealed a diastasis of more than 3 mm in 32/1,000 of the subjects presenting one or the other sign of the disease, and in 64/1,000 of those having clear clinical data. In 1963, de Sèze et al. [320] took a series of 103 patients with rheumatoid arthritis among which they randomly sampled a group of 57 patients showing or having shown clinical cervical signs. Of these 52 were X-rayed in the flexed position, which showed 10 to have atlantoaxial subluxation, i.e. 19.23%. Contrariwise, Serre et al. [316] found a much higher percentage, viz. 38.33% on in-patients. Mathews [233] "found that of 76 consecutive patients seen as out-patients, a quarter had 3 mm of separation or more in lateral tomographs of the neck taken in flexion." Cibert [69], in his thesis, recorded among 475 in-patients of both sexes with rheumatoid arthritis, 25 atlantoaxial subluxations. However, less than half of these patients, or 201, had had X-rays of the neck, and even those only in the neutral position. He recorded a mean frequency of 17.88%. Stevens et al. [336] denombrated 36 atlantoaxial subluxations in 100 in-patients. According to Smith et al. [332], among 962 in-patients 150 were found to have cervical subluxation at one or more levels. Twenty of these 150 patients had evidence of spinal cord or brainstem involvement at the time of admission. Among the remaining 130 patients in whom there was no evidence of neurological complications, they found 91 forward atlantoaxial subluxations. Forward subluxation was considered to be present if a gap of 3.5 mm or more was observed between the atlas and the odontoid process on the lateral X-ray of the neck in flexion." Conlon et al. [75] found that of 333 patients in a rheumatoid group, 295 had symptoms referable to the neck, and 167 showed changes which were thought to be typical of rheumatoid arthritis. The most striking anomaly was the presence of subluxation. This most frequently occurred between atlas and axis; and separation of more than 2.5 mm in females and 3 mm in males was found in no less than 84, i.e. 23% of the whole series. Finally, in our series, about which we gave the details above, we found 78 subluxations in 174 patients (44.8%). We would like to emphasize that the examination was only performed on 174 patients who were selected with regard to the severity of the disease and the clinical signs of cervical involvement. On the whole, it can be said that 6.4% to 44.8% of rheumatoid arthritis cases develop atlantoaxial subluxation. This wide range deserves comment: in in-patients this percentage is 10–36%, and in out-patients it is 25%.

Taking together all cases published, the percentage rises from 17 to 20, and this can be considered as a mean value. This value is far below our own, but this is indisputably due to the fact that we paid special attention to the radiological detection of this condition.

G. Etiology of Atlantoaxial Subluxation

Usually the reports describe the most often encountered characteristics in atlantoaxial subluxation. Indeed, it seems that a peculiar condition may be individualized by taking into account the data of the clinical examination, of the radiology, of the biology, and even perhaps of the therapy.

1. Clinical Data

We consider the following features to be significant: The *duration* of rheumatoid arthritis, which is often more than 5 years. However, Van Kerkhove [365] reports two cases in which atlantoaxial subluxation was the first sign of the disease as early as the first year, and he considers this to be frequent. Though most atlantoaxial subluxations are seen in patients over 50, it seems that the duration of the disease plays a role. Indeed, besides its occurrence in children, most of atlantoaxial subluxations seen before 50 occur in subjects in whom the disease has been evolving for some time – 5 years at least.

Also significant are *features of articular involvement,* especially the important and disabling deformations of some articulations, and almost always involvements of the hands and the feet, but also, in 58% of cases, of the hip. The latter may be uni- or bilateral with usually more or less accentuated acetabular protrusion and, sometimes, important destruction of the femoral head. The peculiar character of these involvements should be stressed: marked inflammations of the adjacent soft parts, important synovial hypertrophy, and, especially, destructive lesions of the ligaments and tendons bringing about multiple articular luxations. The evolutionary stage with regard to Steinbrocker's classification reflects well the severity of the arthritis: 82% of the cases are classified stage 3 or 4. Moreover, from a functional point of view, these patients are more disabled – only four of them are able to work.

The *presence of systemic signs* also accounts for the severity of the disease, for instance subcutaneous rheumatoid nodules, vascularitis, or Sjögren's syndrome.

Aside from the fact that rheumatoid arthritis is more frequent in females, the sex seems to have no influence.

2. Biological Data

These also reflect the severity of rheumatoid arthritis with subluxation. In our material the sedimentation rate is almost always increased to variable degrees. Serology has been found to be positive in 87% of cases, most often at high rates. High percentages of antinuclear antibodies have been noted 8 times, and in six cases L.E. cells were found.

3. Role of Corticosteroids

It is established that atlantoaxial subluxation is mainly seen in cases of arthritis which had been treated with steroids for a long time. This was the case for 63 of our 78 patients. However, since corticotherapy is most often justified by the severity of the disease, the evolution of the disease itself could be implicated. Besides, Cibert [69] recalls that the rise in utilization of steroids coincides with the systematic study of atlantoaxial subluxation in rheumatoid arthritis. Correlations between cause and effect do not seem to have yet been demonstrated. Those who think that treatment with steroids favours atlantoaxial subluxation point out that steroids would act as well by their osteoligamentous catabolic role as by their analgesic action, thus allowing movements of the cervico-occipital joint, the articulations of which, the transverse ligament expecially, are weakened by the rheumatoid disease. Smith et al. [332] do not agree with this theory.

4. Role of Trauma [206, 261]

A trauma occurring in a patient with rheumatoid arthritis can cause a neurological cord compression symptomatology. In some cases, sudden death has been reported. If atlantoaxial subluxation were not known, it would be diagnosed on this occasion. However, it is not possible to know whether this sometimes mild traumatism has provoked a lesion of the ligament, which, in turn, caused subluxation, or whether it has simply revealed an already existing subluxation. The responsibility of the trauma as regards cord compression has been pointed out mainly in some isolated cases where it had provoked major neurological disturbances and even death. In systematic studies, traumas are less frequently reported. In the well-known study of Isdale and Conlon [182] no death is reported to have occurred after trauma in the 38 patients with atlantoaxial subluxations followed-up for more than 6 years, nor in the 59 patients who died during this period.

Case histories of two of our patients with trauma follow:

La... Valerie, a 36-year-old female with grade 4 seropositive polyarthritis for 19 years, was treated for about 6 years with doses of 15 mg prednisolone. Unbearable neck pains, secondary to an 8-mm atlantoaxial subluxation, led to C1/2 arthrodesis, according to Ramadier's technique (Ramadier and Bombart [281]). Lysis of the bone graft had occurred and some stabilization was only due to the metallic loop. In flexion movement, the subluxation was again present but of only 4 mm. Thirteen months after the operation, the patient was in a traffic accident (she was seated in the front seat of a car which was run into from behind, and suffered a whiplash injury). A few hours after the accident she died from internal hemorrhage although no cord compression signs were recorded in the clinical examination. It seems that, despite the imperfect arthrodesis, the intervention played a part.

The second case, *Han... Albertine,* a 73-year-old female presented since 1962 with seropositive grade 4 polyarthritis. From the onset of the disease, she had been treated with 5 mg prednisolone. On the occasion of an arthroplasty of both knees with Shiers' prothesis in 1972, a complete examination was carried out, and X-rays of the neck and of the cervico-occipital joint showed marked upward atlantoaxial subluxation with erosion of the odontoid process (Figs. 53–55). The neurological examination was normal save for an occipital pain in the area of the right greater occipital nerve sequential upon sneezing. Investigations carried out in 1975 showed the radiological changes to be slightly aggravated; and, neurologically, numbness of the left cheek was present. In July 1976, after a fall, a definite pyramidal tract involvement necessitated hospitalization.

Note that a trauma can bring about, besides classical atlantoaxial subluxation, other changes, such as subluxations of the lower cervical spine with compression of the spinal cord, most usually C3 and C4 [206], and also spontaneous spinal epidural hematoma [122]. As concerns fractures of the cervical spine, they occur mainly in a spine stiffened by ankylosing spondylarthritis [153, 341, 369, 389, 404].

Traumas may have different origins: senility, articular deformations secondary to rheumatoid arthritis, and perhaps even preexistent pyramidal tract involvement. Consequently, cord compression signs are not proven to be secondary to traumatism.

Inopportune chiropractic manipulations, and also surgical anesthesia may be considered as traumatisms [261]. Also, movements carried out during intubation may be harmful to the patient. Thus, it is useful to know in advance the state of the cervico-occipital joint and of the cervical spine; the anesthesist must be informed of it, and sometimes the patient must wear a collar.

H. Follow-up Studies in Atlantoaxial Subluxations

To form an opinion on this, we have two studies bearing on large series of patients with a long follow-up. Thus, it is now possible to form an opinion about the natural history of atlantoaxial subluxations. In 1966 Conlon et al. studied 333 patients with rheumatoid arthritis in which they found 23% atlantoaxial subluxations.

The follow-up survey was done 5.5 to 6.5 years after the assessment [182]. In the meantime, 59 patients had died, among whom were 17 with atlantoaxial subluxation, but in none was death secondary to this lesion. As to the patients without atlanto-axial subluxation, death seemed never to be due to rheumatoid involvement of the neck. Among the 171 patients who had a 6-year follow-up, 38 subluxations were found at the first examination and 79 during survey examinations. None of these cases was found to have significant neurological complications, not even those with marked subluxation. Some of the patients with neck symptoms in this series have been helped by simple immobilization by a collar. But most have had no treatment at all, and none has had surgery. According to the authors, "positive evidence of serious complication was not obtained ... In none of those who have died, has death been directly related to the subluxation. For these reasons surgical intervention in the absence of progressive neurological or vascular changes seems unwarranted." Even more striking is the study of Smith et al. [332] which concerns a series of 962 patients comprising 150 atlantoaxial subluxations among which 20 had evidence of neurological complications at the first examination. The 130 patients without spinal cord or brain stem involvement have been followed-up 5–14 years after the first examination, a mean duration of 7.8 years. During this period, only one out of five patients with grade 4 diastasis (more than 8 mm) showed aggravation. Does this mean that as soon as a certain degree of subluxation is attained, it can hardly aggravate? This is indeed our opinion and we think that this finding could be explained by the ankylosis secondary to destructive arthritis in the atlanto-occipital and atlantoaxial joints. In one of the other five patients who initially had subluxation, the subluxation was no longer found at the follow-up examination—even though he was of grade 4. It would be of interest to know whether it was a matter of a subluxation reducible by the radiodynamic study, and what was the state of the articulations between the occiput, the atlas, and the axis. In that case, also, one could imagine that there was no subluxation in the neutral position and that ankylosis of the joints between these three bone parts has brought about ankylosis, thus stabilizing the subluxation.

These authors have also considered the effect of treatment on the evolution of subluxation. Among those who have been usefully wearing a collar, 33% were aggravated from a radiological point of view and 66%

showed no modifications, as concerns the subluxation. These results may be superposed on those obtained in the group of patients who did not wear their collars often enough. As concerns the corticosteroids: "the incidence of atlantoaxial subluxation was approximately equal in both the steroid and nonsteroid treated group. It also appears that forward luxation at C1/2 progressed poorly in patients taking steroids, when compared with similar lesions found in those not receiving this drug. The difference in the progression of subaxial luxations between these two groups was not so marked, but there seemed to be less deterioration among those taking steroids." Forty-six patients died without a follow-up examination. Among the 41 deaths, only one seemed to be due to a lesion of the cord, but the cord or brain stem involvement could easily pass undiagnosed. In our relatively small series of subluxations, only 12 patients have had one or several follow-up examinations during the last 7 years. In these patients, we never saw any improvement of the atlantoaxial subluxation, but in eight cases the diastasis did not progress. Contrariwise, there was, in three cases, an occurrence of progressive upward atlantoaxial subluxation, as has also been recorded by Smith et al. [332]. In our series, death has, to our knowledge, never been due to neurologic lesions of the neck.

As concerns the evolution of the neurological signs in atlantoaxial subluxations, see Part 4, Chapter 2.

IV. Upward Atlantoaxial Subluxation

Theoretically, a luxation or a subluxation is a disturbance of the normal relation of two articular surfaces. Denomination is given with regard to the direction of the displacement of the cranial part. Thus, the condition termed by us "upward atlantoaxial subluxation" should be called "downward atlantoaxial subluxation" or merely "downward atlas subluxation." We have retained the terms "upward atlantoaxial" or "upward odontoid subluxation" because these are the generally accepted denominations. Davis and Markley [89] were the first to report this condition from autopsy findings in a case of fatal medullary compression by the odontoid process projecting into the foramen magnum. In 1958, Storey [339] reported another fatal case of subluxation of the odontoid process into the foramen magnum with backward compression of the spinal cord. Note that the studies of Coste et al. in 1952 [78] reported the radiological signs in atlantoaxial subluxation but did not mention upward displacement of the odontoid process. In 1960 Garcin et al. [138] reported a detailed radioclinical study in a case of "axoidoatlantal invagination"—upward displacement of the axis through the atlas. In 1961, Sharp and Purser [324] and Martel [223], and in 1963 Bland et al. [32], described minor degrees of upward subluxation of the axis. In 1963, Martel and Abell [226] reported autopsy findings in two cases of sudden death in patients with rheumatoid disease due to atlantoaxial dislocation with herniation of the odontoid process through the foramen magnum and compression of the medulla. The ligaments were lax resulting in extreme mobility of the atlanto-odontoid joint, but otherwise the joints were normal. The same year, Serre et al. [316] carried out an exhaustive study on rheumatismal lesions in the cervico-occipital region, and pointed out the striking frequency of "basilar invagination" seen with inflammatory arthritis. In 1968, Webb et al. [390], reported a similar case with post-mortem findings of severe atlantoaxial subluxation;

the odontoid process projecting into the foramen magnum and compressing the medulla. The right lateral mass of the atlas was completely destroyed. Death was due to bilateral thrombosis of the vertebral artery in its upper cervical portion. Newman and Sweetnam, in 1969 [257] recommended a surgical method for occipitocervical fusion. To support this method, they describe a case of upward and backward displacement of the odontoid process with anteroposterior odontoatlantal diastasis. In a survey of 76 cases of rheumatoid arthritis, Mathews, in 1969 [233], found the odontoid process to project beyond the foramen magnum in 5% of the cases. Rana and Taylor, in 1971 [284], reported a clinical case of upward displacement of the tip of the odontoid in rheumatoid arthritis and emphasized the necessity of being aware that the consequences of this lesion may resemble cerebrovascular complications. Surgical treatment of this condition is well established: axial skeletal traction followed by occipitoatlantoaxial arthrodesis with or without decompression of the foramen magnum. Swinson et al. [349] in 1972 reported three cases with different degrees of upward subluxation of the axis through the foramen magnum with posterior neck pain, with or without neurological symptoms. He described the radioclinical follow-up of a case in which an increase of the upward luxation is seen. In 1973, two papers dealt with the surgical technique to be used in upward luxation. Finally, the same year, Rana et al. [283] reported eight new cases, which were radiological incidental findings in patients with cervical pain or neurological signs. The author himself [92, 102] found 12 upward atlantoaxial dislocations among 153 cases of rheumatoid arthritis, i.e. 7.8% of the cases. His criteria are different from Rana's. Indeed, Rana speaks about upward luxation only when the dens is more than 10 mm above the palatosuboccipital or McGregor line, whereas the author diagnoses upward subluxation when the dens is above McRae's line of the foramen magnum, even if only by a few millimeters (Figs. 45–46).

A. Morphologic Changes

Frontal tomograms permit a precise analysis of the morphology of the articular lesions causing upward subluxation. Constant involvement of the atlantoaxial joint was noted either as dislocation or as alteration or even complete destruction and collapse. On the other hand, the condyloatlantal interspaces were only involved in seven cases. The lateral tilting of the skull with regard to the axis of the spine is directly related to the asymmetry of articular destructions (Fig. 49).

This articular involvement is combined with morphological changes of the odontoid process mostly by erosion, and sometimes by hypertrophy.

Sagittal tomograms allow visualization of topographic modifications of the odontoid process with regard to the basion on one hand, and to the atlas on the other. They seem to be more significant for demonstration of upward luxation of the axis (Fig. 47). Besides, half of the cases in the author's series, and only one out of eight in Rana's showed anteroposterior odontoatlantal diastasis. The anteroposterior subluxation is always irreducible, due to multiple articular destructions.

B. Modifications With Regard to the Usual Radiological Landmarks

Several convergent criteria characterize upward subluxation of the atlas (Figs. 45, 48).

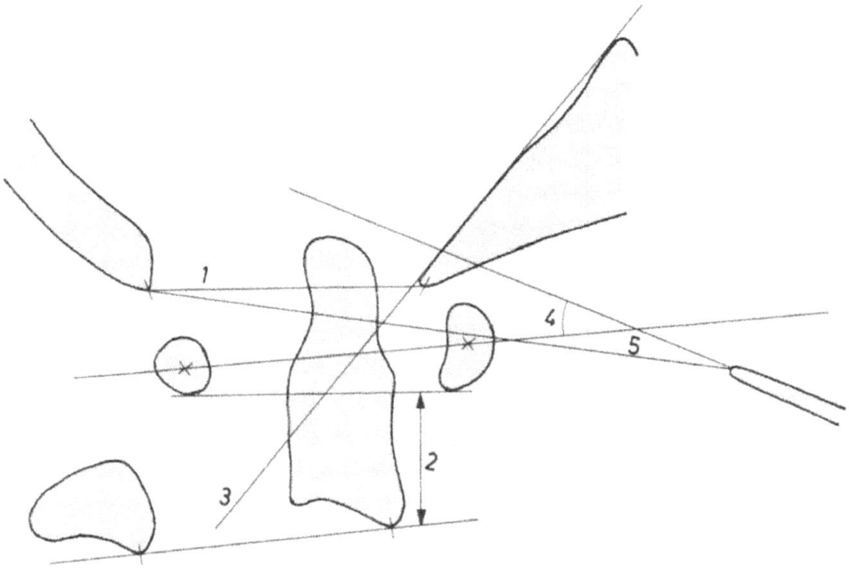

Fig. 45. Usual radiological landmarks in upward atlantoaxial subluxation (downward or caudal atlantoaxial subluxation) in lateral view. *1* McRae's line of the foramen magnum, *2* Distance between the basal plane of the atlas and the basal plane of the axis, *3* Basilar or Thiebaut-Wackenheim-Vrousos's line, *4* Bull's angle, *5* Chamberlain's line

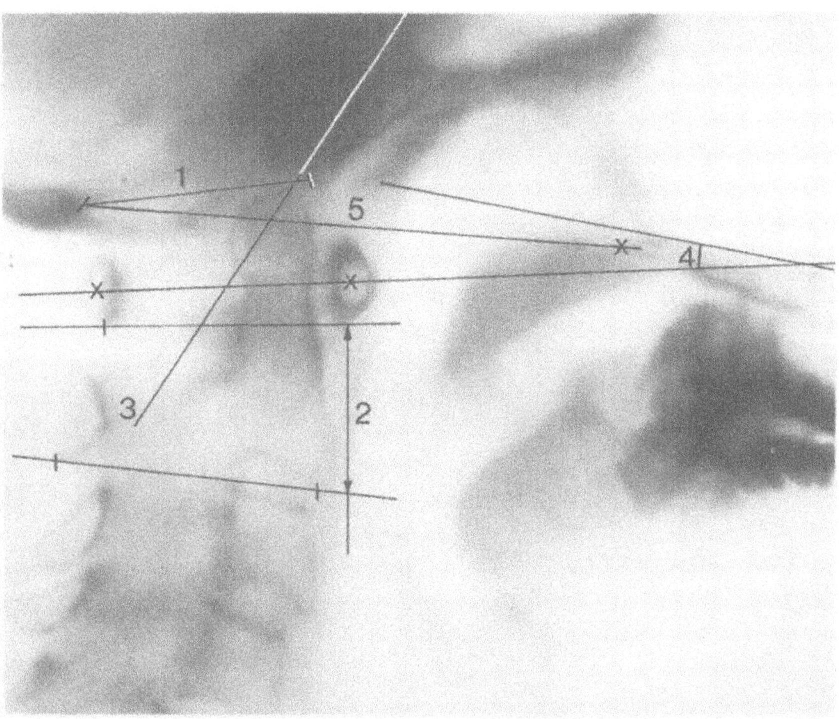

Fig. 46. Example of moderate upward atlantoaxial subluxation, downward or caudal atlantoaxial subluxation in lateral view with the usual radiological landmarks (for numbers see Fig. 45)

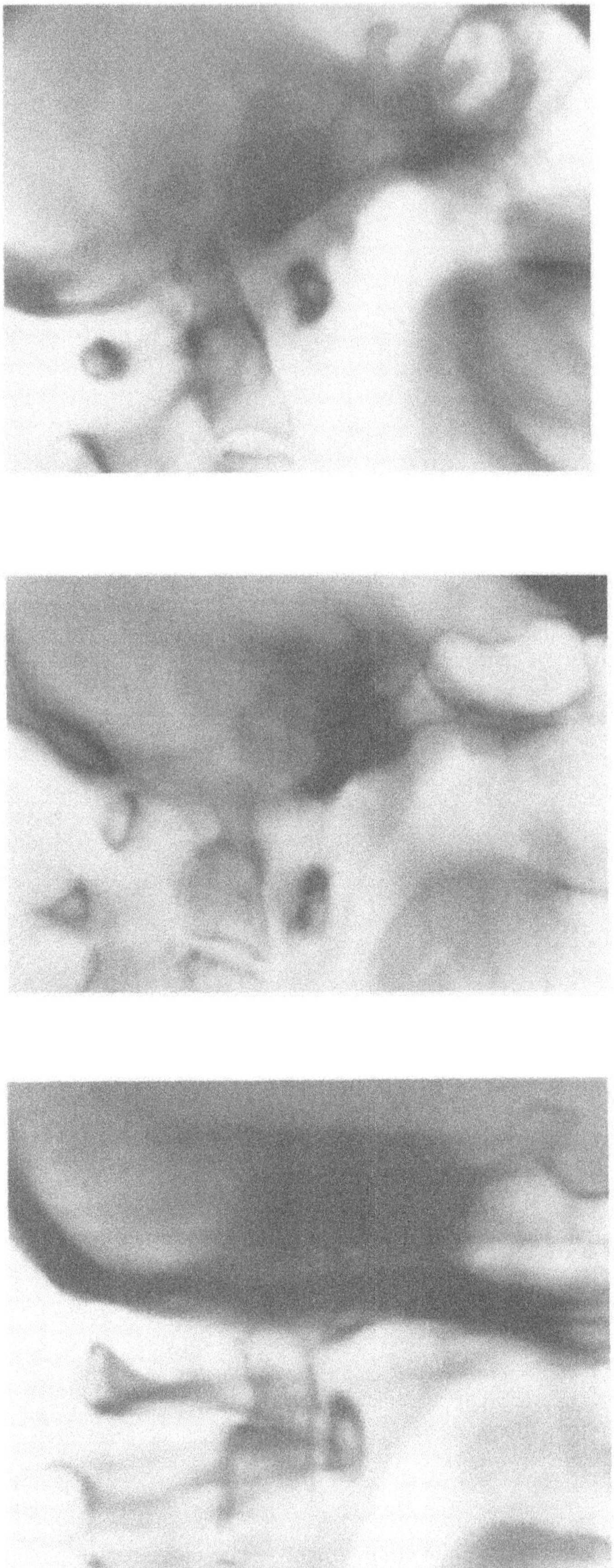

Fig. 47. Three examples of upward atlantoaxial subluxation in lateral view

The tip of the odontoid process lies above the bimastoid line and is level with or above McRae's line of the foramen magnum. The latter landmark is, most of the time, quite reliable but it may be at fault when the odontoid process is eroded or strongly demineralized. The position of the body of the axis, immediately behind the arch of the atlas, in a lateral radiograph of the neck, is then a useful radiographic sign, on plain films as well as on tomograms. The distance between the basal plane of the atlas and the basal plane of the axis depends too much on the height of the axis to be a valuable criterion of upward subluxation.

The tip of the odontoid process is always above the basilar or Thiebaut-Wackenheim-Vrousos line. Under normal circumstances, the basilar line lies at an angle to the posterior aspect of the odontoid tip. In cases with anteroposterior atlanto-dental dislocation, the overlapping of the basilar line is much more marked because of the backward displacement of the odontoid process.

The constantly abnormal Bull's angle leads one to think that anteroposterior tilting of the atlas is associated with upward subluxation, so that this angle can have a negative value.

Other lines of measurement may be useful for diagnosis, for example the bimastoid and bidigastric line in frontal views and Chamberlain's line in lateral views; but the anatomical structures which determine these landmarks are too distant from the odontoid process to be reliable with respect to the smaller displacements.

In fact, upward subluxation should not be defined with regard to lines. It is the association of osteoarticular changes in the cervico-occipital and C1/2 articulations, and of the situation of the odontoid process with regard to McRae's line—either level with or above it—which characterizes this lesion. In atlantodental diastasis, isolated ligamentous lesions may provoke a displacement, whereas in upward luxation articular lesions must always be present. Finally, we would like to point out that if anteroposterior dislocation narrows the spinal canal at the level of the atlas, upward dislocation narrows the foramen magnum (Figs. 47, 53–55).

C. Correlations Between Basilar Invagination and Rheumatoid Arthritis

Great confusion exists about the occurrence of basilar invagination in rheumatoid arthritis owing to the fact that diagnosis was made by means of lines and indexes, while the nature of the lesions determining anatomical changes was disregarded. Some found it to be of 44%, while others added to the confusion by using the term "pseudobasilar invagination."

In conclusion, five conditions are to be strictly differentiated, as follows:

Primary Basilar Invagination

It is quite conceivable that a patient may have at the same time primary basilar invagination and rheumatoid polyarthritis. According to Schmidt and Fischer [311], congenital basilar invagination is present in 1% of the population. Close examination shows the type of primary basilar invagination: anterior basilar invagination with hypoplastic basioccipital (clivus), thin clivus, and platybasia; paramedian basilar invagination with hyperplastic exooccipital, flattened and hypoplastic occipital condyles, and an increased Schmidt's angle; an association of these two types.

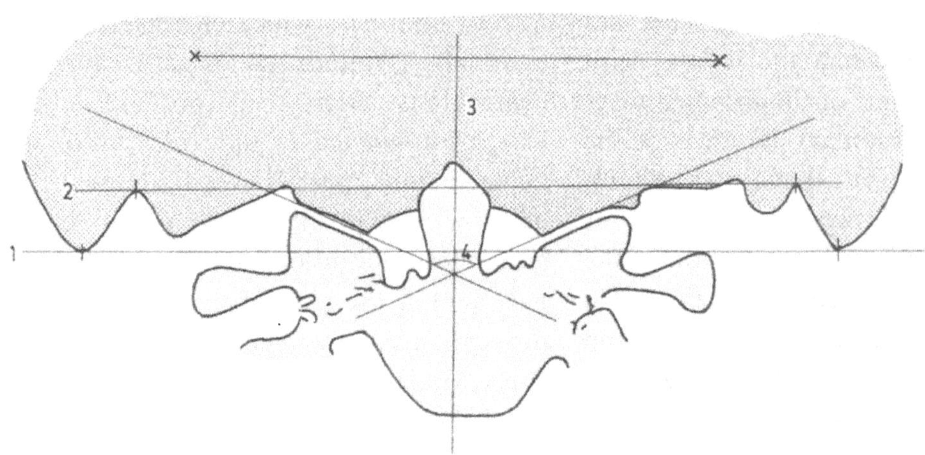

Fig. 48. Usual radiological landmarks in upward atlantoaxial subluxation in frontal view. *1* Bimastoid line, *2* Bidigastric line, *3* Intervestibular line, *4* Condylar angle

Secondary or Acquired Basilar Invagination

This condition is most often seen in osteopathies such as osteomalacia, Paget's disease, and hereditary fragility of the bones. Separate papers deal with this problem in non-rheumatic diseases [101]. It is well known that patients with polyarthritis also frequently have common osteoporosis, sometimes associated with osteomalacia, whereas pure osteomalacia is rare. Osteoporosis in polyarthritis seems to result from different physiopathological factors, e.g., rheumatoid inflammation, immobilization, presenile and senile involution, and corticotherapy. Osteoporosis is not responsible for softening, and, thus, for basilar invagination.

S. Werne, who reported three cases of true secondary basilar invagination, raises the hypothesis of chronic local hyperemia correlated with synovitis of the atlanto-occipital articulations, responsible for secondary demineralization with softening and deformation of the occipital condyles. This type of deformation would be similar to acetabular protrusion during coxitis in rheumatoid arthritis.

W. Martel's Pseudobasilar Invagination [223]

Martel studied the involvement of the cervico-occipital joint in rheumatoid arthritis and described a case of pseudobasilar invagination, i.e. a case with no invagination of the edge of the foramen magnum. In fact, it was not only a matter of erosion of the lateral masses of the atlas and of the occipital condyles—changes also recorded by us—but also of erosion of the tip of the basioccipital. Indeed, these changes modify the classical landmarks, and especially the basal angle formed between the clivus and the anteroposterior diameter of the foramen magnum (Boogard's angle, described in 1865, is no longer used [42]), but do not produce basilar or even pseudobasilar invagination properly speaking. However, the measurement of the length of the basioccipital (3.2 cm $\pm$0.3, according to Schmidt and Fischer), and the study of its morphological modifications, should be part of the radiotomographic study of the cervico-occipital joint in rheumatoid arthritis.

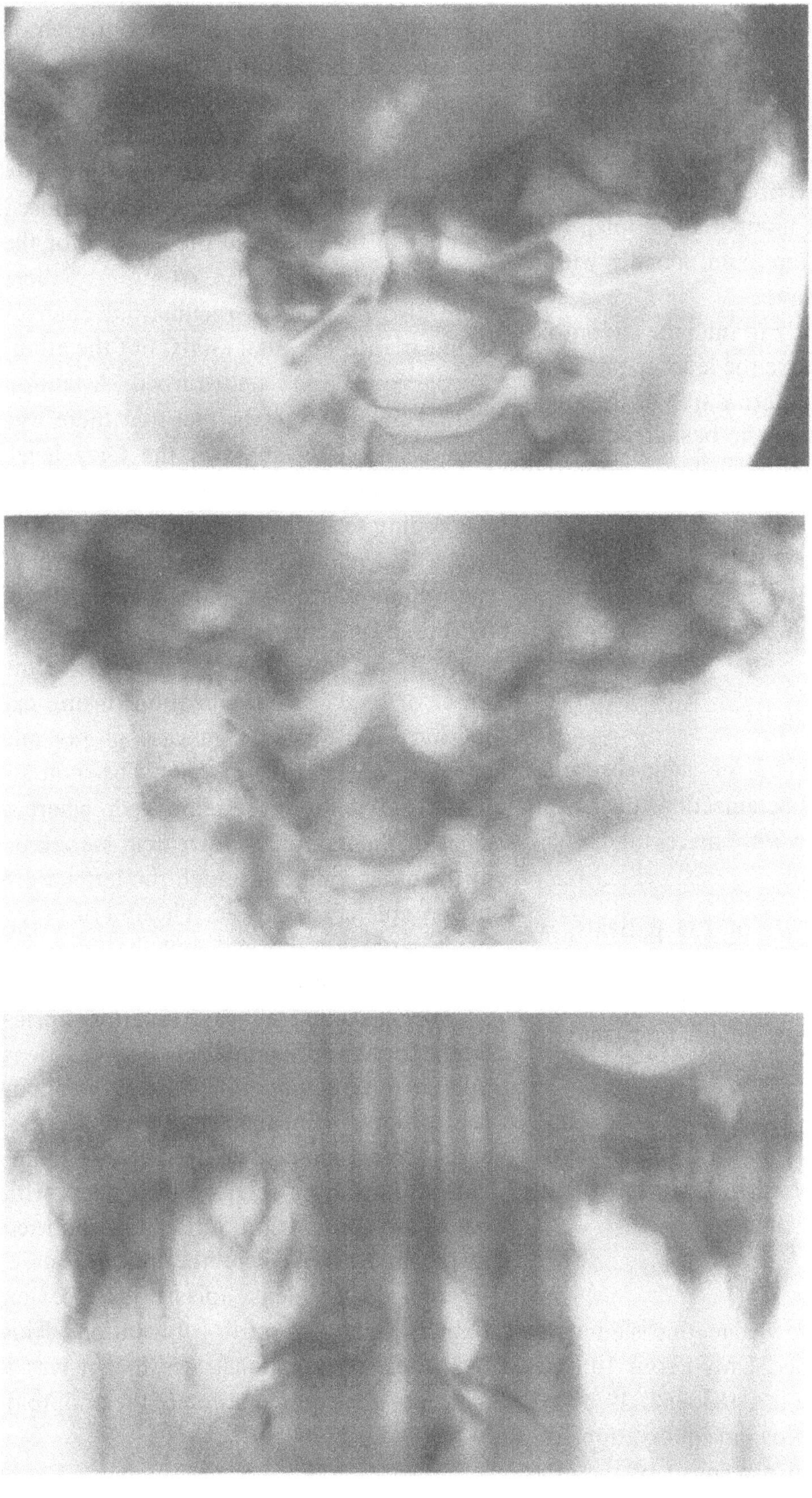

Fig. 49. Three examples of upward atlantoaxial subluxation in frontal view. Pictures correspond to the same cases in Fig. 47

Wackenheim's Congenital Supra-atlantal Extension of the Odontoid Process [380]

This congenital condition occurs with two variants. In the first, the odontoid process lies not only above the level of the superior margin of the anterior arch of the atlas but also above Chamberlain's line, and above the basilar line, and actually within the foramen magnum.

In the second variant, the odontoid process extends above the level of the superior margin of the anterior arch of the atlas, but lies tangential to the basilar line as in cases with a normally developed odontoid process.

It goes without saying that mineralization and articular surfaces are normal in this congenital malformation.

Upward Luxation of the Odontoid Process

This lesion would be the main cause of modifications in the connections of the cervico-occipital joint with the skull base in rheumatoid arthritis.

In our own series of 153 patients, we found three mild primary basilar invaginations and 12 upward luxations of the odontoid process, but no secondary basilar invagination or pseudobasilar invagination.

V. Backward Subluxation of the Atlas

To the author's knowledge, this is an extremely rare occurrence. Only about 10 cases have been reported [83, 183, 368, 393, 401].

Backward atlantoaxial subluxation consists in posterior displacement of the atlas on the axis. In rheumatic diseases without congenital anomalies, this displacement may only occur in the following circumstances: destruction of the anterior arch of the atlas, pathological fracture, or destruction of the odontoid process.

Four times it was a lesion of the odontoid process, and, in Verjaal and Hardner's [368] case, the X-ray of the neck disclosed absence of the odontoid process and of the anterior arch of the atlas. At autopsy, there were also destructive rheumatoid changes in the atlanto-occipital joints, but the atlantoaxial joints were undisturbed. Attention should be drawn to the fact that there was also a soft tissue mass at the C1/2 level, which was felt to be a contributing factor. According to the authors, there was no evidence that allowed the presence of a rheumatoid nodule to be excluded, rather than, as stated, of a meningioma.

We have had the opportunity to see the onset of backward subluxation during extension of the head in a case of juvenile chronic polyarthritis (Fig. 61). The right atlantoaxial joint was undamaged, whereas signs of rheumatoid involvement were seen at the other joints, although the latter were not completely destroyed. The anterior arch of the atlas was normal, but the odontoid process was almost entirely destroyed.

Wackenheim [380] gave functional principles for the differentiation between dens aplasia and fracture of the base of the odontoid process with an unstable pseudofracture. Unfortunately, no functional examinations have been carried out in cases with backward subluxation of the atlas reported in the literature. As to the author's case, it reacted like dens aplasia, i.e. flexion reduced the backward subluxation. This functional sign demonstrates that it was a matter of an acquired lesion of the odontoid process.

VI. Backward Subluxation of the Occiput

To the author's knowledge, only a few cases with this type of subluxation have been accurately reported. Coste et al. [80] reported the first to occur in ankylosing spondylarthritis, which they called "forward atlanto-occipital subluxation."

Tomograms of the neck show a backward subluxation of the occiput causing spinal cord compression. The atlantoaxial joints have become loose, so that the posterior arches of the atlas and of the axis almost obturate the foramen magnum. Unfortunately, no functional X-rays were performed. The displacement was probably an acquired condition, since a lateral film of the neck, which had been taken 21 years earlier, was normal.

Another case, reported by Walcher et al. [387], concerns a rheumatoid arthritis evolving over 17 years. The articular surfaces of the atlanto-occipital joint have lost connection. The odontoid and anterior arch of the atlas are situated under the inferior aspect of the clivus and seem to raise the latter. The tip of the odontoid lies 21 mm above the palato-occipital line of Chamberlain. Besides, there exists a dehiscence (spina bifida) of the posterior arch of the atlas, so that it may be a matter of a congenital malformation. McRae [241] had already evoked this possibility.

Chapter 6 Other Radiological Investigations

I. Angiography

A. Arteries

The *vertebral artery* arises from the first part of the subclavian artery. It ascends through the foramina in the transverse processes of all cervical vertebrae save the seventh, and begins the V4 and V5 segments. When it leaves the axis, the vertebral artery runs toward the transverse foramen of the atlas while describing a first vertical curve with inward concavity. It issues from this foramen and curves backward behind the lateral mass of the atlas, the second curve being horizontal and anteriorly concave. Then, it pierces the dura and enters the skull through the foramen magnum. The two vertebral arteries may be of unequal caliber, and if so, the left vertebral artery is wider than the right. Normal variations in the course are described, as well as abnormal courses in congenital malformations of the cervico-occipital region.

The *extramedullary arterial* system has multipleorigins. There exists as many arteries entering the spinal canal as there are cranial nerves. Thus, the vascularization is segmental and directed transversally with regard to the great axis of the spinal cord. Three groups of arteries form this network: the anterior spinal arteries, the posterior spinal arteries, and the lateral spinal arteries.

Anterior Spinal Arteries

The two *anterior spinal arteries*—the left and the right—arise from the vertebral arteries a little bit behind the point where the latter join to form the basilar trunk. They descend in front of the medulla oblongata, and unite on the midline to form the anterior spinal trunk.

Posterior Spinal Arteries

The two *posterior spinal arteries* arise from the vertebral arteries just behind the anterior spinal arteries, and run immediately along the posterior aspect of the medulla oblongata and the spinal cord. Each of them divides into two branches which descend vertically.

The lateral spinal arteries or radicular arteries approach the spinal cord laterally. At the level of the neck, they arise from the vertebral artery and from the ascending cervical artery. Each of them enters the intervertebral foramen along with the corresponding nerve and divides by following both roots. When they reach the cord, they divide into ascending and descending twigs.

Vertebral angiography is of little interest in rheumatic diseases. Subluxations occur progressively, and displacements of bones are quite small, so that, thanks to their elasticity, the arteries adapt easily to modifications in their course. Moreover, two conditions can favor pathological changes in the arteries, i.e. a brisk subluxation or collapse of the C1 and C2 vertebrae, and common

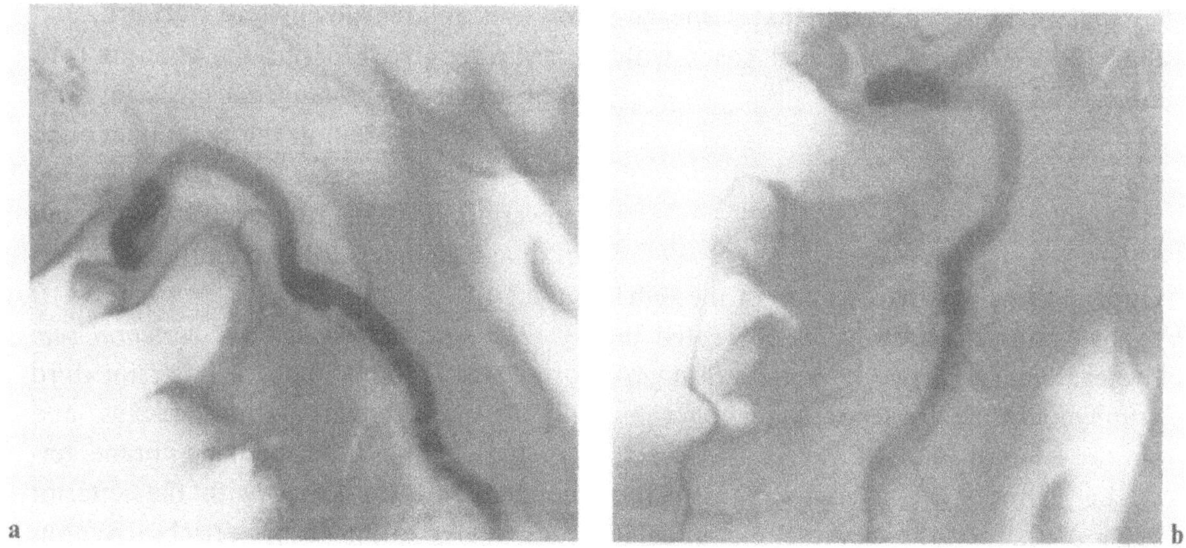

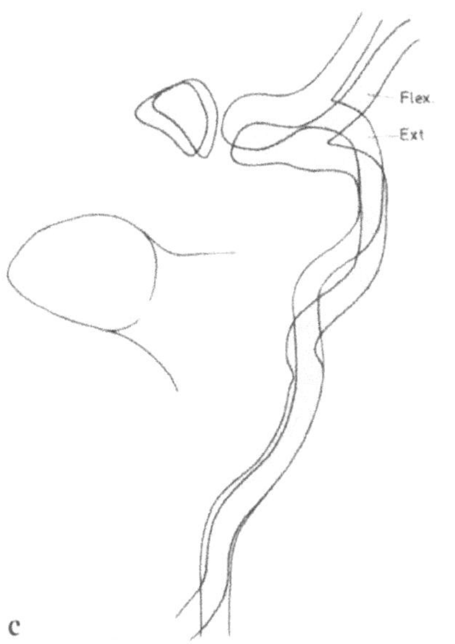

Fig. 50 a–c. Vertebral arteriography in a case of anterior atlantoaxial subluxation. **(a)** Extension. **(b)** Flexion. **(c)** Diagram of both previous positions

osteoarthritic changes in a patient with severe arthropathy. Let us recall that, from a neurological point of view, the symptoms of vertebral artery insufficiency are well known, and that they lead, systematically, to the indication of vertebral angiography. This was the case with two of our patients, both with rheumatoid arthritis and C1/2 reducible subluxation. Moreover, one had multiple spondylitis of the cervical spine. The vertebral angiography was normal in both cases (Fig. 50). Indeed, even angiographic projections, carefully performed in different positions of the head – flexion, extension, and rotation – did not show evidence of any significant arterial anomaly, and especially of changes in the blood flow and in the caliber of the arteries. We did not extend this investigation to a larger number of patients since it had been negative in the two who had definite neurological symptoms.

Let us, however, recall that some authors [83, 390, 399] described cases with arterial lesions.

B. Veins

Our experience in opacification of the veins in the occipito-vertebral area is limited to five examinations, two by vertebral angiography and three by cervical phlebography via the femoral vein.

Let us recall the normal pattern of the veins of the occipito-cervical region, as it has been reported by Wackenheim and Braun [383a] in their monograph (Fig. 51).

Venous drainage in the cranio-cervical area is supplied by two systems: a main one by the internal jugular vein and a secondary one by the vertebral vein and its principal afferent branches. Both systems are abundantly anastomosed both in depth and in other more superficial regions (Figs. 51 and 52).

The internal jugular vein, due to its caliber, is the most important drainage channel in the cranio-cervical area. It originates opposite the jugular foramen at the confluence of three principal sinus channels:

The lateral sinus in its sigmoid section
The superior petrous sinus
The inferior petrous sinus

The vertebral vein is formed on both sides by the confluence of the two principal components of the venous roots. These roots form, on the one hand, the anterior root or anterior condylar vein and on the other hand, the posterior root of the vertebral vein.

The anterior root of the vertebral vein is represented by *the anterior condylar vein* which originates at the level of the junction of the anterior third and the medial third of the perioccipital venous plexus. It follows an oblique downward, outward, and forward course, crossing the anterior condylar canal and joining the posterior root of the vertebral vein in the exocranial area. The anterior condylar vein, still called the prevertebral vein, represents the second drainage channel in the cranio-cervical region.

The posterior root of the vertebral vein originates at the level of the posterior third of the perioccipital venous plexus and crosses the atlanto-occipital membrane, terminating in confluence with the anterior root to give origin to the vertebral venous system.

Numerous *anastomotic channels* exist between the different systems. They are represented by superficial and posterior anastomoses, and deep and anterior anastomoses.

The *superficial and posterior anastomoses* are made up essentially of mastoid emissary veins which unite the lateral sinus to the external jugular vein systems and to the vertebral venous system, anastomosing with the posterior root of the vertebral vein.

The *deep and anterior anastomoses* are, for the most part, made up of posterior condylar veins which only variably (in about one-third of cases) originate at the level of the jugular foramen. They course downward and backward, anastomosing with the vertebral venous system at its origin.

In our five examined cases, we did not observe any pathological changes in the venous system in the cervico-occipital region. Let us emphasize the fact that this technic allows one to demonstrate the whole venous system in the cervico-occipital region as well as in the lower cervical spine. Thus, phlebography is specially indicated in cases of diffuse cervical myelopathy to dis-

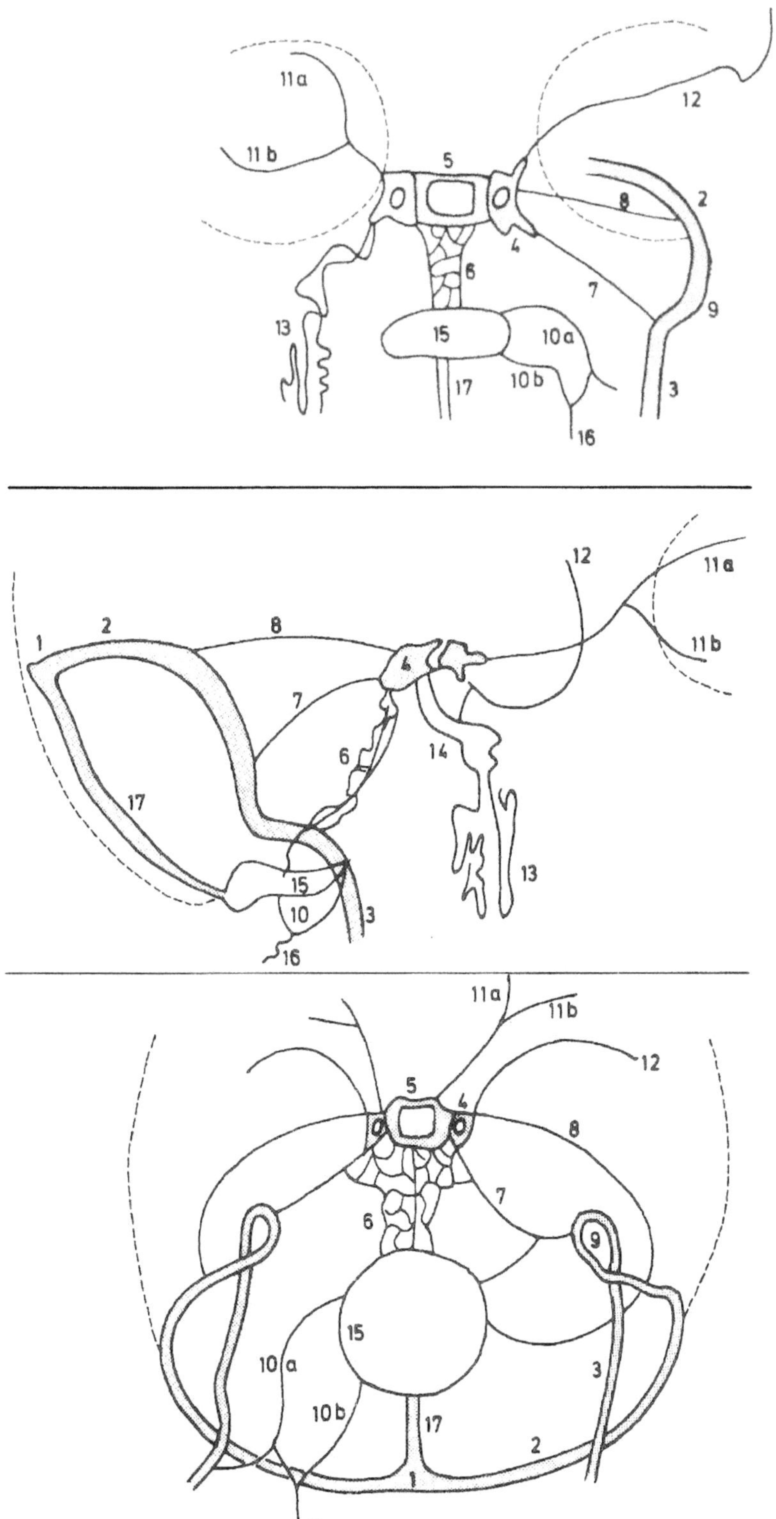

Fig. 51. Drawing of the main venous sinuses. *1* Torcular, *2* Lateral sinus, *3* Jugular vein, *4* Cavernous sinus, *5* Coronary sinus, *6* Clival plexus or basilar plexus (Virchow), *7* Inferior petrous sinus, *8* Superior petrous sinus, *9* Jugular groove, *10* Anterior *(a)* and posterior *(b)* condylar veins, *11* Superior *(a)* and inferior *(b)* ophthalmic veins, *12* Fronto-parietal sinus (Brechet), *13* Pterygoid plexus, *14* Pterygoid veins in the foramen ovale, *15* Foramen magnum plexus or perioccipital plexus, *16* Vertebral veins, *17* Occipital sinus (inconstant)

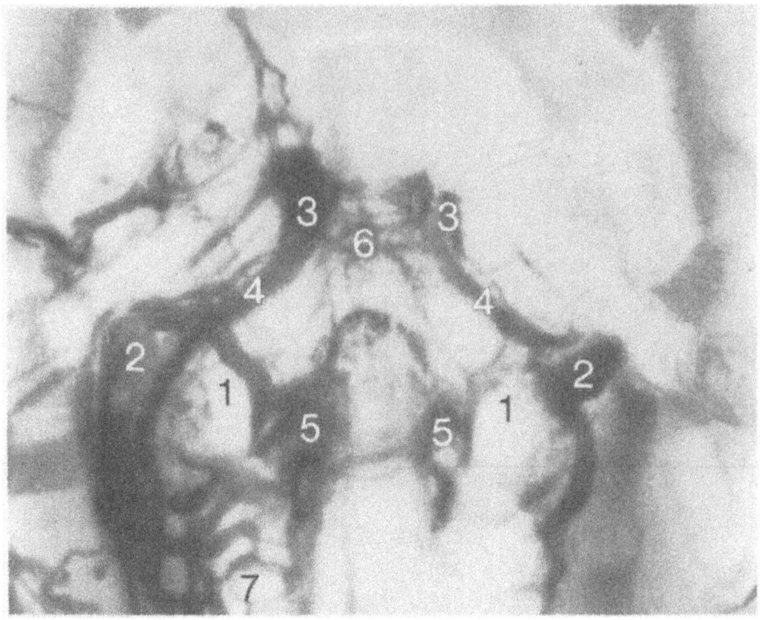

Fig. 52. Phlebography of cervico-occipital region by femoral route in axial projection. *1* Anterior condylar vein, *2* Jugular vein, *3* Cavernous sinus, *4* Inferior petrous sinus, *5* Intraspinal plexus, *6* Transverse occipital sinus, *7* Anastomotic plexus. (Courtesy of J. Théron, Caen)

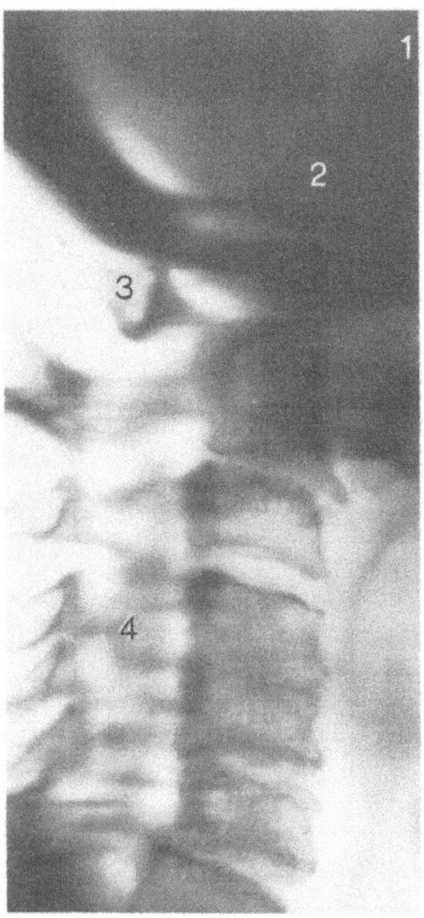

Fig. 53. Gas myelography demonstrating normal spinal cord between C2 and C7 *(4)*, narrowing at level of C1 *(3)*, and insufflated fourth ventricle *(1)* through the foramen of Magendie *(2)*

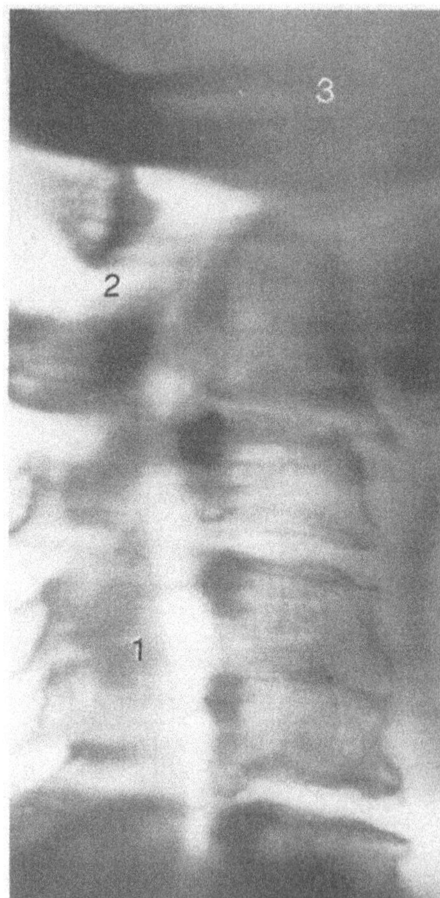

Fig. 54. Arrest of the gas column at the level of the body of the axis in the anterior subarachnoidal space *(2)*. This space is normal below *(1)*. No insufflation of prebulbar cistern *(3)*

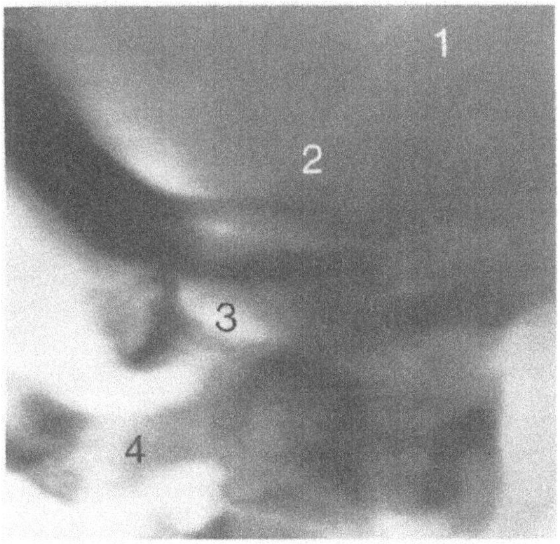

Fig. 55. Normal passage of gas in fourth ventricle *(1)* through foramen of Magendie *(2)* and considerable narrowness of the posterior subarachnoidal spaces at the level of C1 *(3)*. These spaces are normal below *(4)*

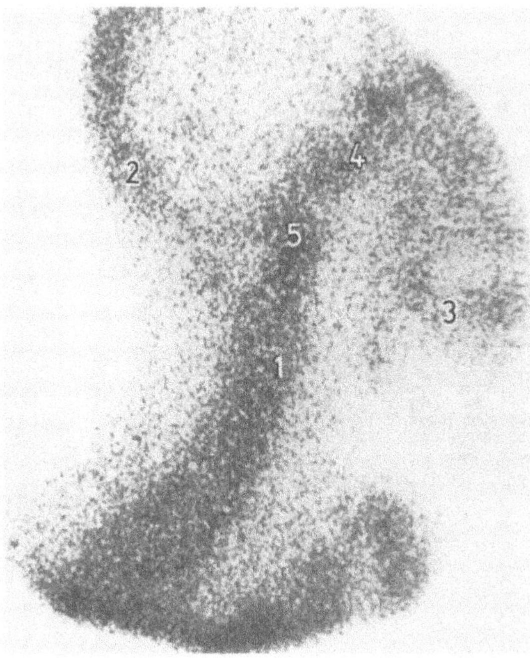

Fig. 56. Bone scanning with pyrophospate ^{99m}Tc. Lateral view of the cervical spine *(1)* and of cervico-occipital region *(5)*. *2* Occipital squama, *3* Mandibule, *4* Basilar process

tinguish upper and lower cervical lesions. We will devote a future study to this subject.

II. Myelography

Lesions of bones and their incidence in the spinal cord may be definite enough to justify surgery without preliminary contrast medium investigations—vertebral angiography or myelography. The latter performed with gas or with positive contrast is indicated in very precise circumstances: first, suspicion of spinal cord atrophy entailing absence of compression of this thinner cord, and second, suspicion of spinal cord compression despite moderate stenosis of the canal. In this latter case, myelography may be performed to provide evidence of a possible thickening of the intracanalicular soft tissues [159]. Finally, cases with very advanced or diffuse lesions—cervical or cervico-occipital—or with two major lesions, one in the upper and the other in the lower segment, justify myelography in order to define the location of the pathogenic area (Figs. 53–55).

III. Bone Scintigraphy

Numerous authors perform arthroscintigrams, but only J.M. Bastin [23] has reported results in the cervico-occipital joint.

We had the opportunity to perform bone scintigrams in 20 patients with rheumatoid arthritis.

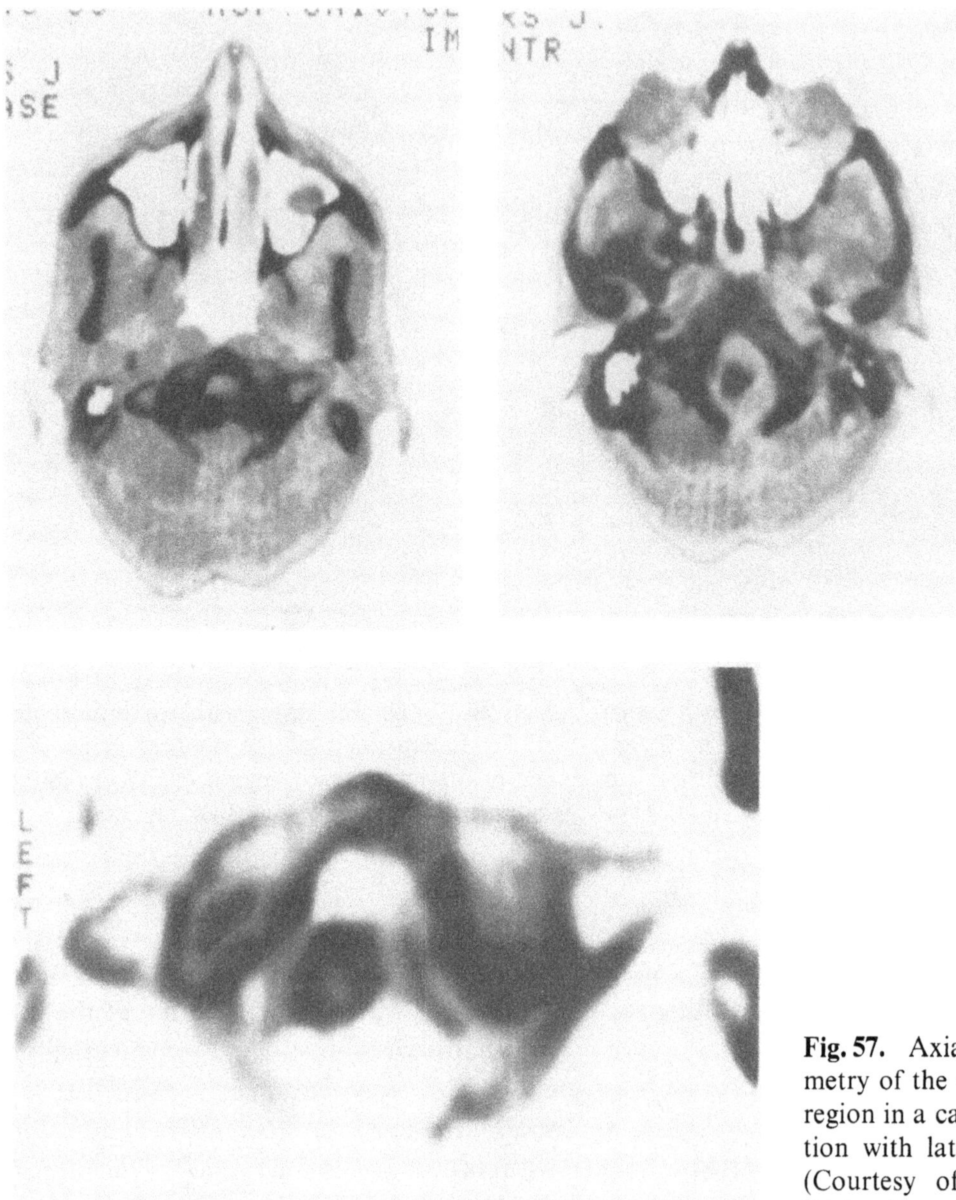

Fig. 57. Axial tomodensitometry of the cervico-occipital region in a case of malformation with lateral dislocation. (Courtesy of D. Baleriaux-Waha, Brussels)

Technique. Intravenous injection of 10 μCi pyrophosphate labelled with technetium-99m. Scanning is done 4 h later by means of a gamma camera equipped with an omniview system; it comprises a view of the whole body and complementary localized views. (The phosphated compound sets on the bone by a similar mechanism as tricalcic phosphates.) The fixation rate does not reflect the total amount of mineral substance contained in the bones but its turnover. It goes without saying that pathological features are seen in arthritis only insofar as there is involvement of the juxta-articular bone. Interpretation of scintigrams in this area is particularly difficult. On lateral scintigrams, the petrous and the mastoid portion of the temporal bone are projected close to the cervico-occipital joint, and may be confused with it. Moreover, the line of the spinous processes and the vertebral canal are poorly defined. On a posterior view, the vertebral bodies are poorly individualized in the cervical segment, contrary to the lumbar segment.

Results (Fig. 56). We have not observed hyperfixation in the craniocervical joint compared to the cervical spine, nor signs of localized hyperactivity. And yet, all 20 patients examined complained of pain in the neck and had atlantoaxial subluxation. Besides, scintigraphy of the entire body showed several hyperfixation foci in the peripheral articulations.

This negative result may be interpreted differently, thus:

The modifications in the juxta-articular bone are not significant enough.

The articulations of the cervico-occipital joint are hidden by bone structures which have a high affinity for pyrophosphates, whereas they have themselves only a poor affinity.

In spite of clinical and radiological signs, lesions in the cervico-occipital joint have none or a non-significant development.

IV. Computerized Axial Tomography

This new radiological technic will provide investigations in rheumatic disease of the cervico-occipital joint without harm to the patient. Although, it is too early to go into this procedure. Figure 57 illustrates the technic.

Part 6 Radiology in Other Chronic Inflammatory Rheumatic Diseases

Chapter 1 Juvenile Chronic Polyarthritis

Though chronic rheumatism in children was already well documented, Still's original and semiologically accurate description [337] threw new light on this condition, then termed Still's disease.

The french pediatric school and R. Debré describe two forms of chronic rheumatism in children: (1) *Still's disease,* occurring in early childhood with predominantly synovial changes, a severe course, involvement of the general status, diffuse amyotrophy, and, finally, cachexia and death. This description is most certainly erroneous since the prognosis is usually fairly good, though fatal forms have been reported, (2) *ankylosing and deformative chronic polyarthritis* with cessation of statural growth and intermittent fever.

Other pediatricians have less definite views, and admit the possibility of transitional forms, some even of a unique type. Up to recent years, French rheumatologists, in agreement with the specialists of other countries, are of the latter opinion.

Generally accepted is the classification of Bywaters et al. based on their long-term follow-up (25 years) of 217 cases examined initially, at a very early stage of the disease. In 1975, at the 8th European Rheumatology Congress in Helsinki, Bywaters et al. [55] proposed the following classification:

Definite juvenile chronic polyarthritis (JCP), a synonym for Still's disease. Onset of the disease before the age of 16, with involvement of four or more joints for a minimum period of 3 months. The disease is seronegative (no gamma-M rheumatoid factor). It is polyarthritis with more or less systemic disease or pauciarticular involvement, frequently associated with chronic iridocyclitis. There may also be some cases of systemic disease with onset in adult age.

The following joint involvements must be excluded:

Juvenile rheumatoid arthritis. Onset before the age of 16 of a disease with IgM rheumatoid factor, frequently associated with nodules, vascular lesions, and characteristic erosions on radiographs of the hands and/or the feet. Prognosis as in rheumatoid arthritis in adults

Juvenile ankylosing spondylitis. Onset of disease before the age of 16 with involvement of joints of the lower extremity occurring before involvement of the sacroiliac joints or of the spine

Psoriatic arthropathy (as in adults)

Polyarthritis associated with ulcerative colitis or Crohn's disease (as in adults)

Polyarthritis associated with other disorders such as systemic lupus erythematosus, familial Mediterranean fever etc.

This classification could be used for epidemiologic studies but is also of interest for the study of the cervico-occipital joint.

If cervical involvement is so frequent in children that, according to some, it represents one of the major diagnostic criteria, cervico-occipital joint involvement is much more rare, and the actual frequency of

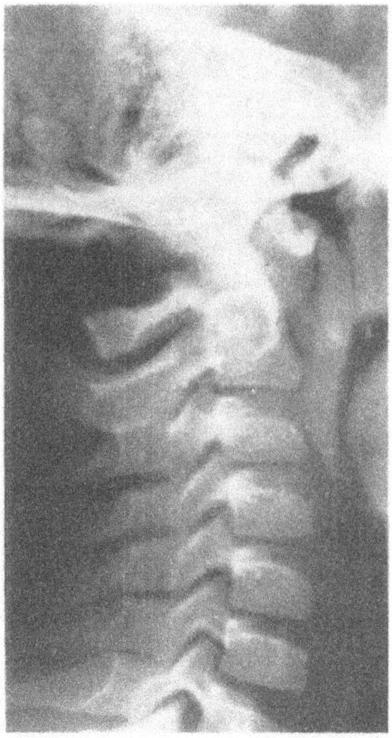

Fig. 58. Atlantoaxial dislocation: this uncommon feature of Still's disease occurred at the age of 7. (Courtesy of J.R. Mann and W. Tempowski, Birmingham)

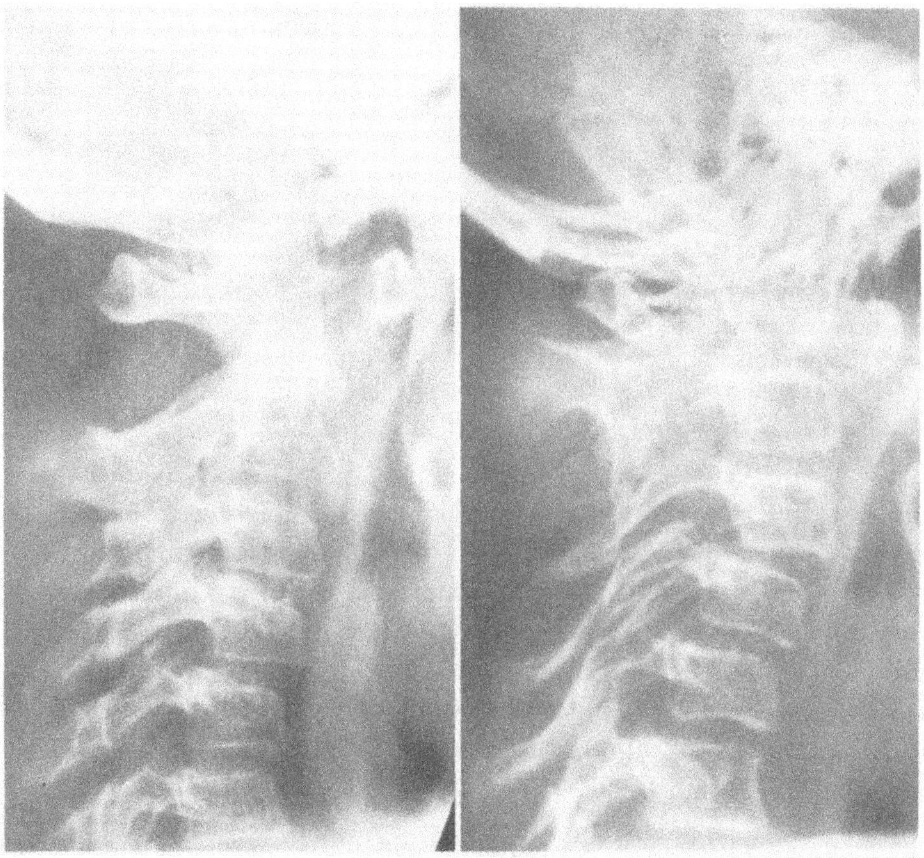

a b

Fig. 59 a and b. Onset of seropositive juvenile arthritis in 1959, at the age of 7. Severe generalized disease. Early atlantoaxial subluxation with bony fusion of apophysal joints of C2 and C3 seen in 1965 X-ray film **(a)**. Further deterioration in the atlantoaxial site and a lower subluxation in 1971 **(b)**. Courtesy of B. Ansell, Taplov)

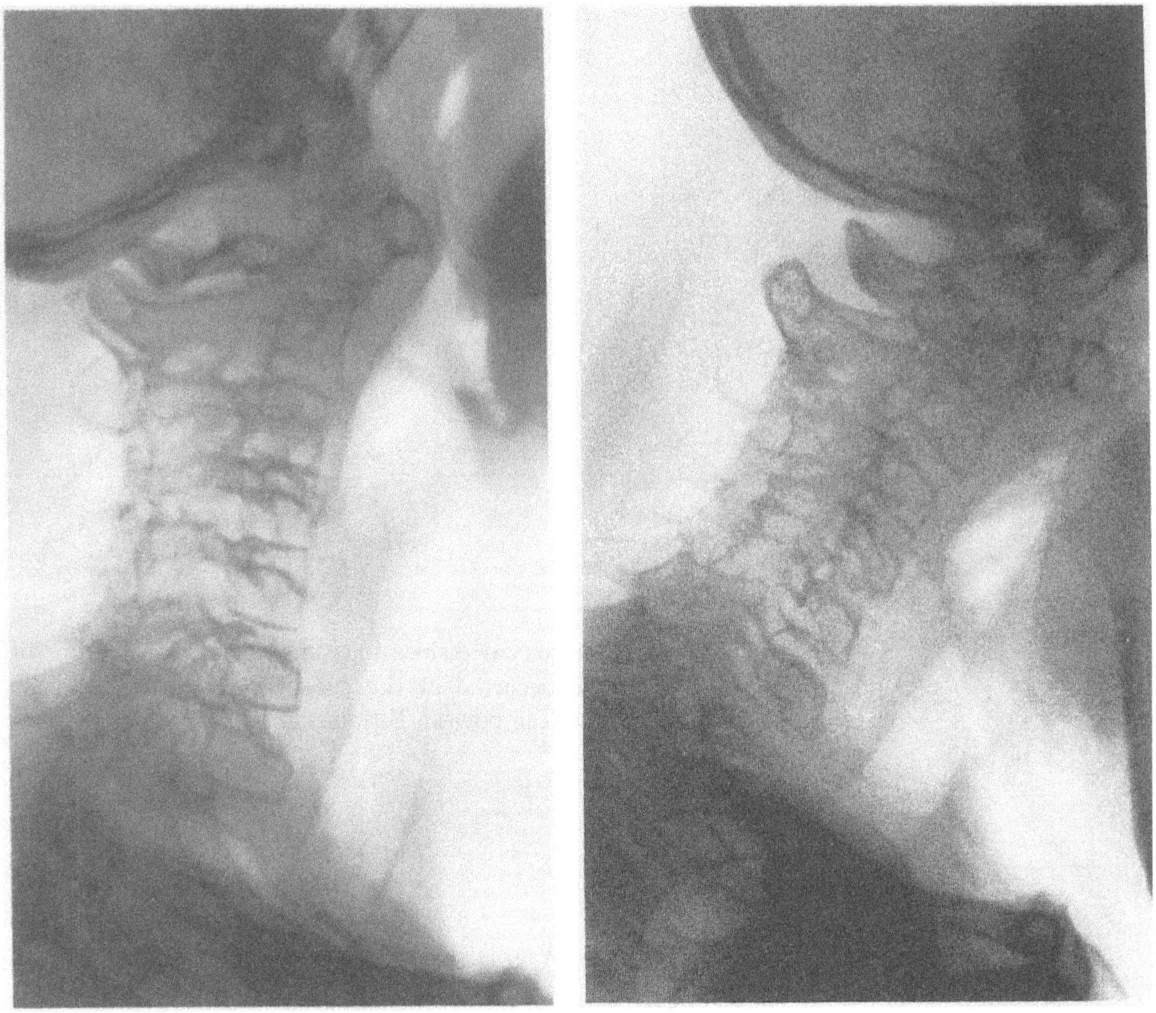

Fig. 60. Seronegative chronic juvenile polyarthritis. Onset at age $2^1/_2$. Corticosteroid treatment. Multiple epiphyseal necrosis (wrists and hips). Child is aged 10 at present. She is 1.04 m tall and her weight is 13 kg. Several joints are affected by polyarthritis. The cervical spine shows a marked demineralization, atlantoaxial diastasis, and fusions between the posterior articulations of C2 to C7. (Courtesy of U. Steiger, Basel)

atlantoaxial subluxation is unknown (Figs. 58–60). The same is true with other types of changes: arthritis, destructions, and new bone formation. Taking into account the confusion in terminology, it is often difficult to classify earlier cases within the categories of the current classification, so that a retrospective study is impossible. Moreover, the changes may pass undetected in childhood and are often only disclosed in adults (Figs. 39, 61, 62).

The peculiarity of the cervico-occipital joint involvement lies in its occurring in a growing skeleton. Perturbations of growth by chronic polyarthritis will be the more important the younger the patient and the more severe the course. Growth disturbances of the limbs or of the cervical spine are determined by several simultaneous and contradictory factors:

A general non-specific factor, linked with the repercussions of the chronic disease, inhibiting bone maturation

A local factor that would cause acceleration of maturation in the involved joints

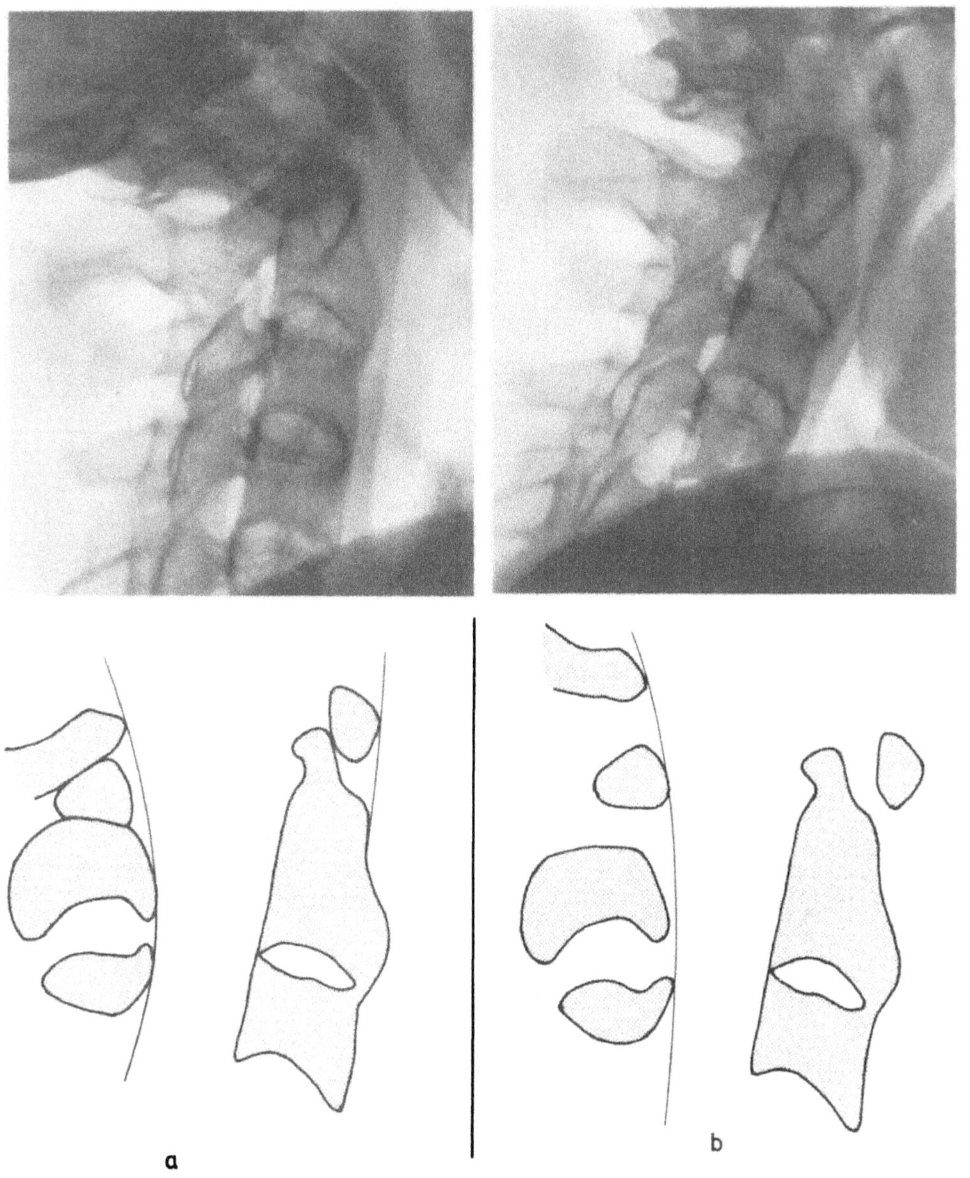

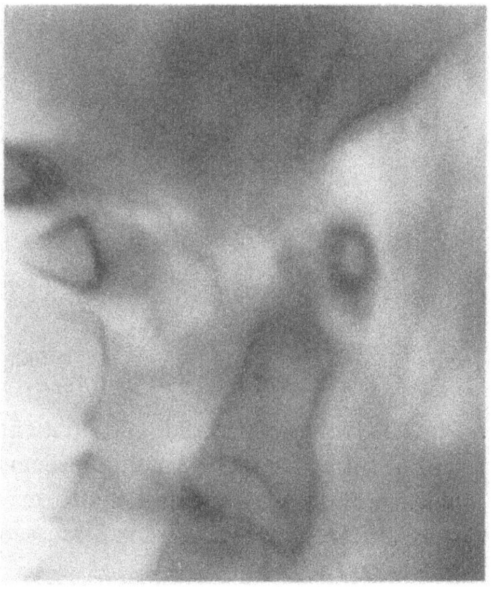

Fig. 61. (a) and **(b)** Flexion-extension movements of the cervical spine take place only in cervico-occipital hinge and are very limited. Almost complete destruction of the odontoid process permits slight backward subluxation of the atlas in extended position of the head. Indeed the anterior aspects of the anterior arch of the atlas and of the body of the axis are abnormally aligned in the extension position of the head, whereas a more or less correct alignment is seen in flexion. Changes in the lower cervical spine are similar to those due to ankylosing spondylarthritis, but in this 34-year-old patient, whose juvenile chronic polyarthritis began at the age of 10, the sacroiliac joints appear normal. **(c)** Tomographic section in the subluxated position showing the markedly eroded odontoid process

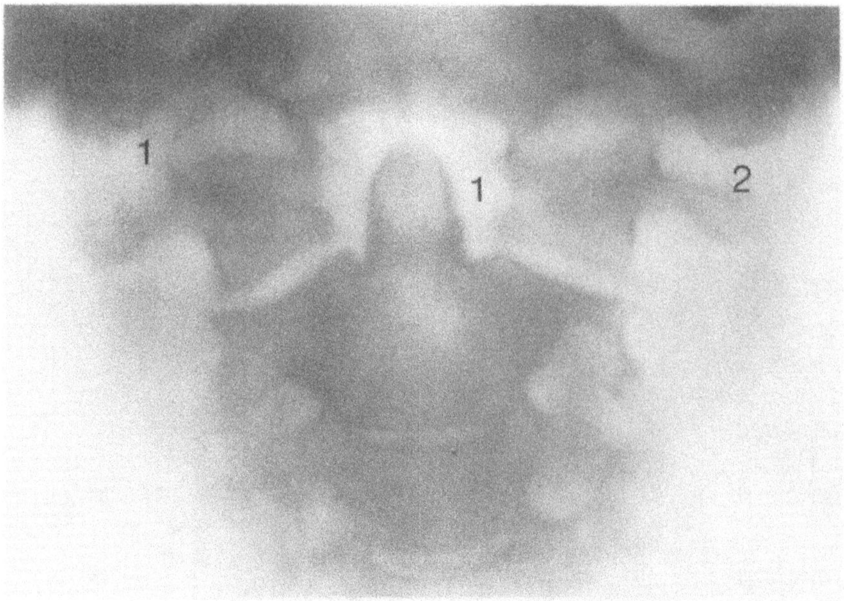

Fig. 62. Bilateral occipitoatlantal arthritis *(1)* in an adult whose juvenile chronic polyarthritis began at the age of 3. Note malformed paramastoid process especially on the left side *(2)*

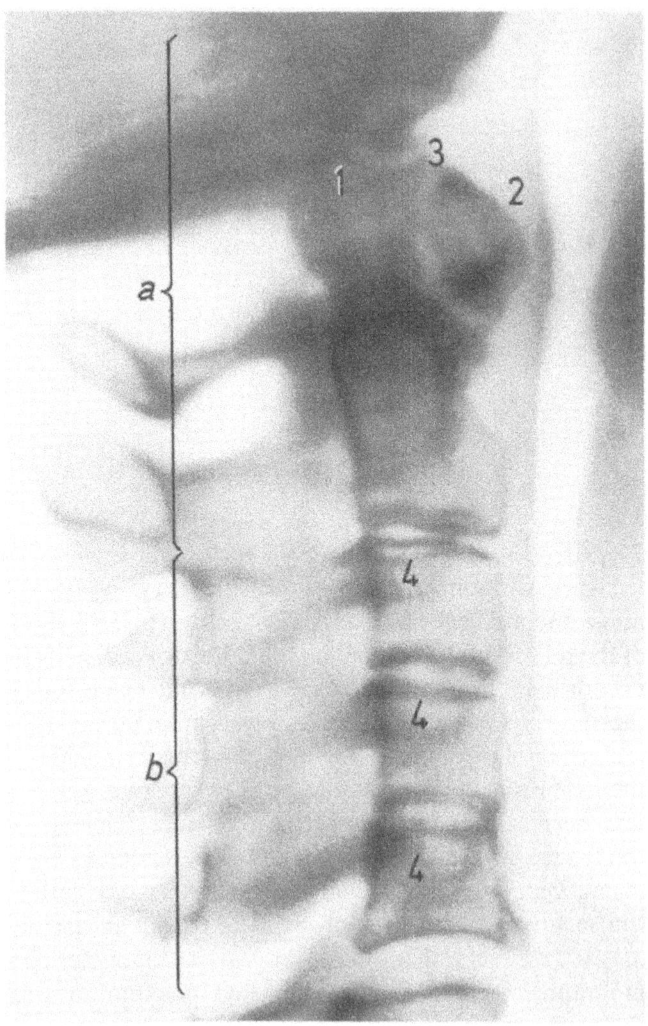

Fig. 63. In this 28-year-old patient with Still's disease everything seems consistent with congenital malformation. Different hypotheses are discussed in the text

Periosteal bone apposition modifying the morphology of the bones

Arthritis, also modifying the morphology of both bones and articular interspaces

Changes occurring in a case of juvenile chronic polyarthritis (Fig. 63) are interpreted with regard to the above criteria. In this case, arthritis of the cervico-occipital joints determined hypertrophy of the clivus, the odontoid process, and of the atlas. A clivodental articulation is constituted, whereas the atlantodental articulation is eroded, the hypertrophic anterior arch of the atlas being embedded in the odontoid process. On the other hand, there is hypoplasia of the C3, C4, and C5 vertebral bodies and disks. The spinal canal is widened at this level and there is bony ankylosis of the posterior apophyseal joints. This is a quite unusual case, not so much as concerns the cervical vertebral block, which is a trivial finding in juvenile chronic polyarthritis, but with regard to the modifications of the bones in the cervico-occipital region. Numerous so-called congenital malformations may be due to ossification disturbances depending on the notochord (hemivertebrae, vertebral blocks, etc.). Wackenheim [380] proposes the term chordopathy for diffuse ossification anomalies and especially for cases with both hyper- and hypotrophic segments, as for instance, the above-described case.

However, we would like to point out that this case of juvenile rheumatoid arthritis showed many other rheumatoid involvements so that three possibilities should be discussed: (1) association of a congenital malformation, (2) cervical localization of the rheumatoid disease, or—a more sophisticated mechanism—(3) the rheumatoid disease producing developmental disturbances of the bones:

Association of polyarthritis with congenital malformation of the spine is only possible with hypotrophic dysmorphoses (i.e. block vertebrae) and is readily recognizable.

Both the hypotrophic changes in the middle cervical spine and the hypertrophic dysmorphosis in the upper cervical spine are due to rheumatoid disease, but this alteration in the morphogenesis cannot be explained.

Since the precise onset of polyarthritis is unknown in this case, one may presume that the disease interfered with and influenced the development of the vertebrae and the disks as other congenital malformations would do. In this hypothesis, the term chordopathy may be adopted but with the adjective "rheumatic."

In any event it should be mentioned that the same disease, i.e., juvenile chronic polyarthritis, can induce both growth arrest and increased growth in an involved segment.

Chapter 2 Ankylosing Spondylarthritis

Atlantoaxial subluxation occurs much more frequently in rheumatoid arthritis than in ankylosing spondylarthritis. However, the first case of upper cervical spine involvement in chronic inflammatory rheumatisms, which was reported in 1933 by Stammers and Frazer [333], concerned ankylosing spondylarthritis. Only much later—in 1951—was a similar involvement described in a case of rheumatoid polyarthritis [89].

In 1944, Rand [285] reported a case of ankylosing spondylarthritis with atlantoaxial subluxation. In 1955, Margulies et al. [222] reported a case of spontaneous dislocation of the atlantoaxial joint in rheumatoid spondylitis with quadriplegia that regressed after laminectomy and surgical fusion from C0 to C4. In 1952, Kornblum et al. [198] reported two cases of ankylosing spondylarthritis with atlantoaxial subluxation. The same year Voluter and Werner [375] also described a case, and Brocher [52] reported two cases. In 1960 Coste et al. [80] published a case of cord compression caused by a rather exceptional lesion—backward occipitoatlantal subluxation. In 1957 Sharp and Purser [324] recorded a series of 10 cases and in 1961 another of 12 cases. In 1961, Martel [223] described erosive lesions in the bones of the cervico-occipital joint, as well as atlantoaxial and atlanto-occipital articular involvement. The next year, he selected 32 cases of severe ankylosing spondylarthritis among which he found five atlantoaxial subluxations. Larger series were published in 1963 by Schilling et al. [308], and by Serre et al. [316]. Finally, in 1967, Hohmann and Walcher [177] attempted to explain the lesions in the cervico-occipital joint during ankylosing spondylarthritis by means of radiodynamic studies.

Ankylosing spondylarthritis preferentially involves the spine. But why should the craniocervical joint be less often involved than in rheumatoid arthritis? According to some, the peculiar embryologic origin of the first two vertebrae would account for this lesser frequency. As a matter of fact, in our opinion it seems much more logical to explain this difference by the anatomic conformation of the articulations. In the cervico-occipital joint, these are of the same type as the peripheral articulations, i.e., diarthroses. In order to support this hypothesis, we tried, in our cases and in those of the literature, to distinguish the purely spinal ankylosing spondylarthritis, i.e., involving only amphiarthroses and diarthro-amphiarthroses, from that involving the peripheral articulations. In these two groups, we noticed no difference in frequency of cervico-occipital joint involvement. However, our series (48 patients) is too small to allow any statistical conclusions. Another argument against our hypothesis is the involvement by an even purely spinal ankylosing spondylarthritis of the posterior interapophyseal articulations, which are also diarthroses. Thus, the type of articulation alone does not account for the relative rarity of involvement of the cervico-occipital joint in ankylosing spondylarthritis. In most anatomicopathologic reports, ankyloses are seen to extend to the atlanto-occipital articulations. Frankel [134, 135] demonstrated that mobility persists at the C0/1 level, the atlantodental articulations and C2/3. According to Forestier et al. [130], the last articulation to be involved would be the atlanto-occipital. Brocher [52] described a case in which the syndesmophytes involve the axis, whereas the joints of the cervico-occipital region are spared.

Our 54 cases of ankylosing spondylarthritis were studied in the same way as the cases with rheumatoid arthritis. The radiological examination was not as easy because of the spinal changes. More or less severe kyphosis is commonly associated with cervical hyperlordosis or forward projection of the head. Owing to that, the plane of the frontal tomograms may not be perpendicular to Reid's line. These distortions have to be taken into account for a correct analysis of the films.

I. Materials

Fifty-four examinations of the neck were carried out in 48 patients—42 males and 6 females. At the time of examination 18 were less than 30 years old, 12 less than 40, 7 less than 50, 8 less than 60, and 9 were over 60. Three patients were grade 1 (presyndesmophytic), 26 grade 2 (florid), and 14 were grade 3 (terminal). In 11 patients an exact determination of the grade had not been possible, so we classed 6 of them as grade 1–2, and the 5 others as grade 2–3.

II. Rarefaction of Bone

If immobilization plays a role in the osteoporosis, this should be more marked in ankylosing spondylarthritis than in rheumatoid arthritis, the spine being then often completely ankylosed. This seems indeed to be true, since among our 54 patients 36 had severe rarefaction of bone. It should be mentioned that its appreciation is rather difficult and very subjective, since precise densitometric investigations are difficult to perform in this area.

III. Articular Changes: Arthritis

This type of lesion seems to be quite exceptional in ankylosing spondylarthritis. Narrowing of the articular spaces, erosions, destructions, and articular ankyloses may be seen. In the series of Serre et al. [316], comprising 29 patients with ankylosing spondylarthritis, the upper articulations were involved only in 2 cases out of the 13 in which they were readily visible; in one case, involvement was bilateral. The lower articulations were found to be involved in 3 of the 18 cases in which they were studied. There too, it was a matter of narrowing and condensation of the interspaces, once associated with osteophytosis. In one case, the interspace had almost entirely disappeared. In our material we have found 8 with atlanto-occipital and 3 with atlantoaxial arthritis.

IV. Destructive Bone Lesions

The destructive bone lesions are quite similar to those seen in rheumatoid arthritis.

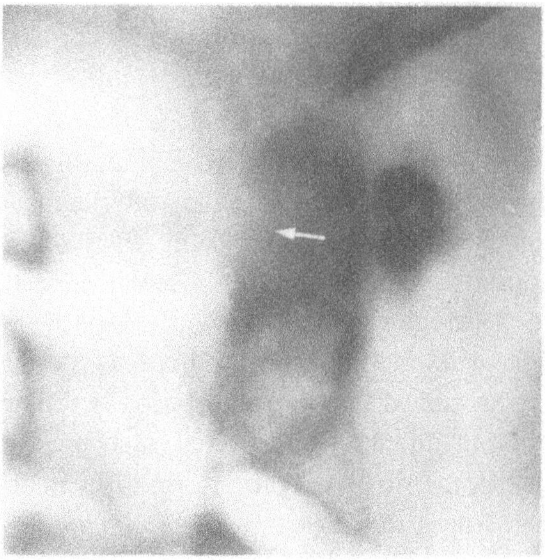

Fig. 64. Blurred posterior aspect of odontoid process in the region of the syndesmo-odontoid joint in a patient with ankylosing spondylarthritis

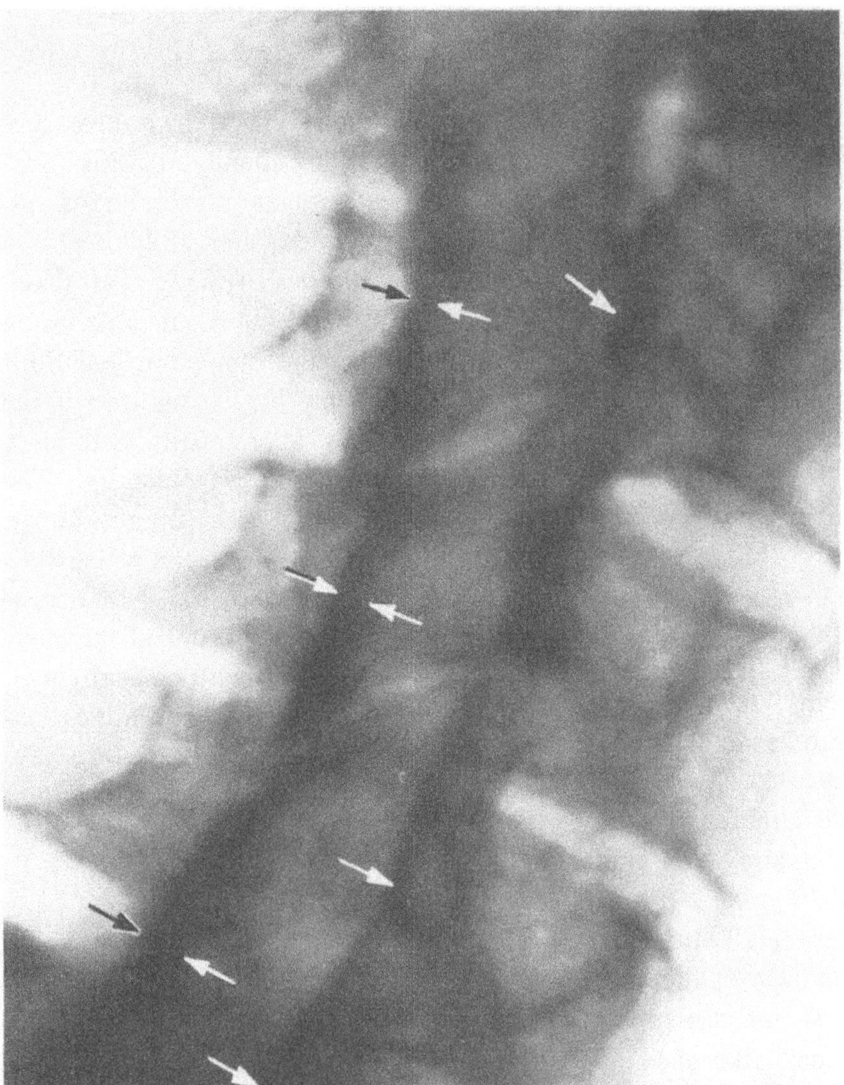

Fig. 65. Calcification of dura in a case of ankylosing spondylarthritis with progressive quadriparesia

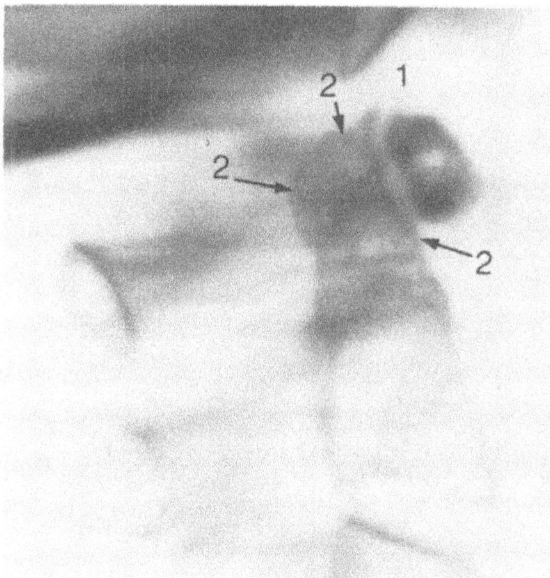

Fig. 66. Shining odontoid with translucencies *(2)* and hyperostotic spicules *(1)* in ankylosing spondylarthritis

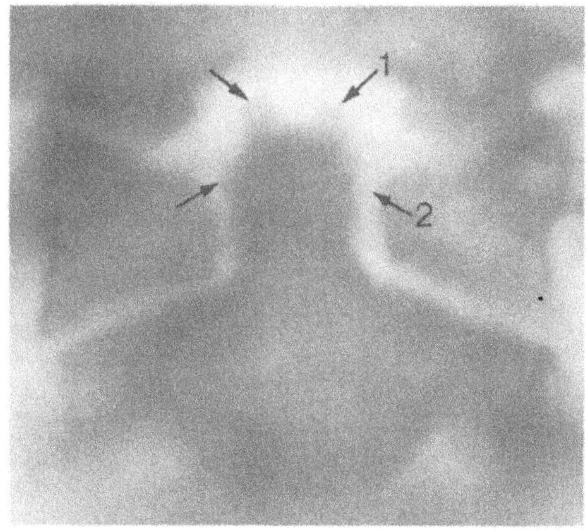

Fig. 67. Hyperostotic horned odontoid *(1)* with hyperostosis of lateral aspects *(2)* in ankylosing spondylarthritis

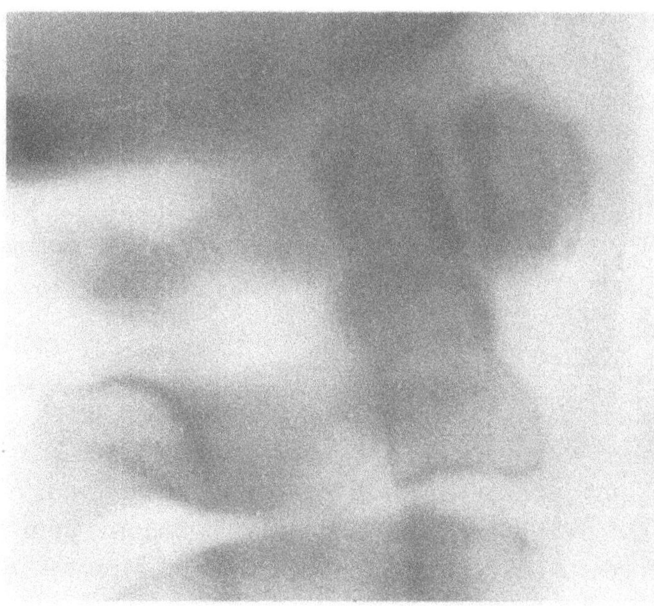

Fig. 68. Hypertrophic and hyperostotic anterior arch of the atlas in a case of ankylosing spondylarthritis

According to Schilling et al. [310], spondylitis of the odontoid process is a common finding. There may be blurred contours and superficial erosions of the dens, but most often the posterior aspect of the dens is eroded (Fig. 64). Schilling et al. have seen these lesions to be always associated with atlantoaxial subluxation, and they record 3 grades as follows:

Grade 1: discrete modification of the shape of the dens and worn-out contours

Grade 2: tapered odontoid

Grade 3: simultaneously, anterior, posterior, and even superior erosion of the dens

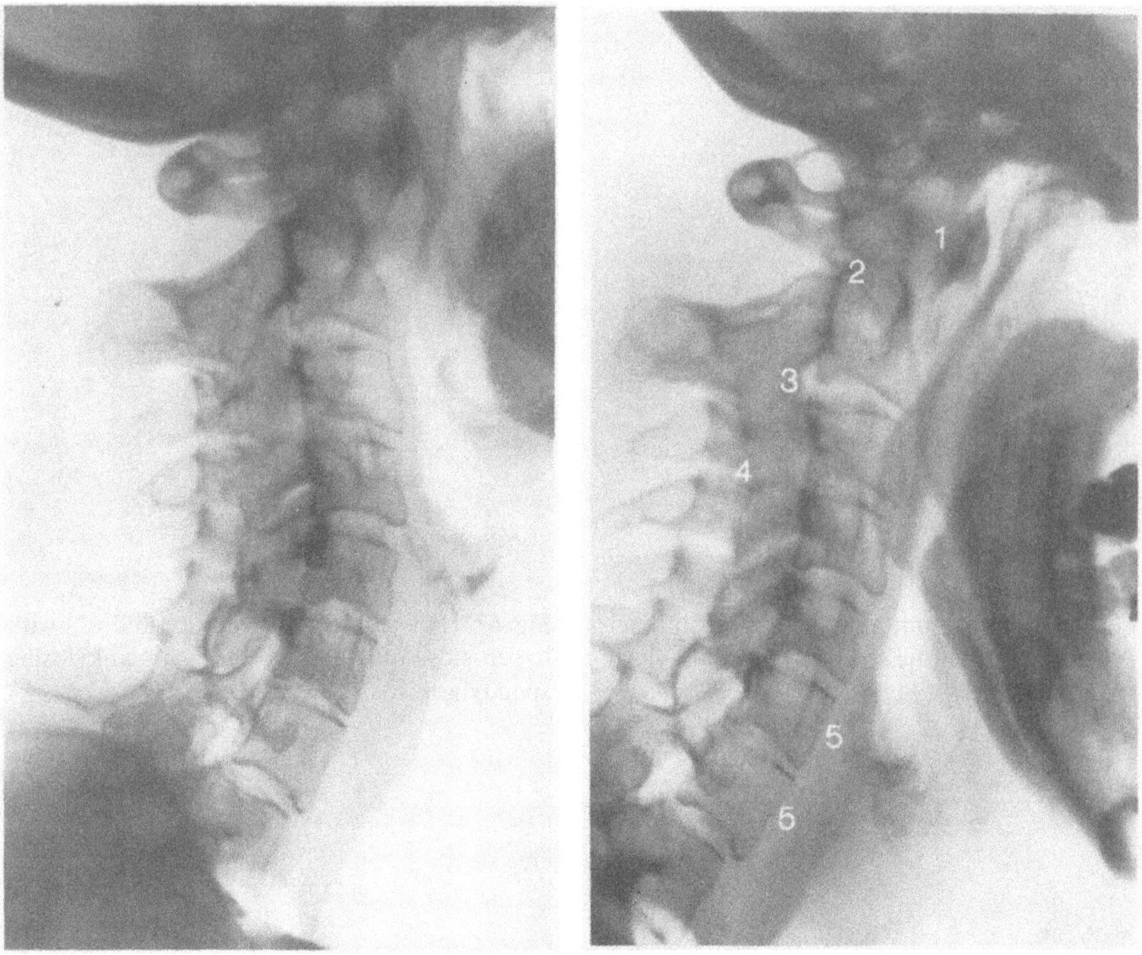

Fig. 69. Atlantoaxial subluxation in neutral position accentuated in flexion, in ankylosing spondylarthritis *(1)*. Posterior encroachement *(2)*, C2–C3 kyphosis *(3)*, fusion of posterior articulations *(4)*, squaring of the C6 and C7 vertebral bodies *(5)*

Superior erosion brings about visible diminution of the size of the odontoid process, and is interpreted as acroosteolysis. Some cases are known with total lysis of the dens. A case of fracture of the odontoid process has been reported by Hohmann [176] and termed by him "fatigue fracture." In this author's opinion, such a fracture would result from ankylosis of the atlanto-odontal articulation in the presence of mobile atlantoaxial articulations.

Destruction of the anterior arch of the atlas, the occipital condyles, the lateral masses of the atlas, and of the upper articular processes of the atlas may also be seen. Another type of destruction is observed at the level of the posterior arch of the atlas. Dorsal kyphosis causes hyperextension of the neck and of the cervico-occipital joints; this extreme position causes atrophy by compression. This condition is reminiscent of the lumbar interspinous arthrosis described by Baastrup.

V. Constructive Bone Lesions

Diminution of mobility in the cervico-occipital joints is very frequent in ankylosing spondylarthritis, but it is not always caused by radiologically visible bone ankylosis. Hohmann surveyed the evolution of the disease and noticed, first, limitation of mobility in the atlanto-occipital joints and only later in the atlantoaxial. There is never only limitation in the latter; the adjacent articulations are always involved.

A. Ossification of the Ligaments

[98, 177, 222, 223, 305, 320]

Despite the marked reduction in mobility, very few pictures of ligamental ossification have been reported. This is surprising in a disease in which the ossifying phenomena are predominant. Only a few cases have been reported to have ossification of the ligaments in the cervico-occipital joint such as the anterior longitudinal ligament, the anterior atlanto-occipital ligament, the apical ligament of the dens, and the alar ligament. Ossification of the posterior atlanto-axial ligament, which is in fact the upward prolongation of the interspinous ligament, has also been mentioned. However, we have never seen ossification of the atlanto-occipital ligament.

B. Ossification of the Meninges

In two of our cases of ankylosing spondylarthritis, lateral X-rays of the neck showed evidence of intracanalar ossifications (Fig. 65). The anterior one forms a linear opacity along the posterior aspect of the vertebral bodies to which it clings in toto, making them thicker. It forms bridges at the level of the disks and stretches from the axis to C7. A meningeal ossification is readily distinguished from a ligamentous one. Indeed, when the meninges are ossified, all radiographic projections determine two parallel linear opacities close to the walls of the spinal canal. On the contrary, ossifications of the ligaments – either anterior or posterior – are visible on lateral projection, and not at all or only poorly on oblique and frontal projections.

The first of our two cases was admitted to a hospital after a trauma, and was seen to have ankylosing spondylarthritis involving both sacroiliac joints and the whole spine. He developed progressive quadriparesis. The prevertebral syndesmophytes were very discrete at the cervical level and the interapophyseal articulations were free, save for C2/3. Intracanalicular ossifications spread as anterior opacities from the postero-inferior aspect of the axis to C7. As to the posterior ossification, it seemed to begin at the median part of the spinous process of C2. The cervico-occipital hinge seemed to have been spared.

The second patient had been complaining for more than 10 years of rachialgia, especially in the upper cervical spine, and of a marked stiffness. Both his sacroiliac joints were involved by ankylosis and the thoracolumbar spine resembled a bamboo stick. The presence of reflex disturbances, e.g., unilateral Babinski and abnormally brisk osteotendinous reflexes, affirmed the existence of a pyramidal syndrome of the lower limbs. Lateral X-rays of the cervical spine showed, as in the previous case, opaque ossifications resembling anterior and posterior laminae, because of the tangential projection of the opacity. The first one is flattened against the posterior aspect of the vertebral bodies; the second is situated at a small distance from the posterior wall of the spinal canal.

Since 1838, when Key described the ossification of some spinal ligaments, 40 such cases have been reported, most of them by

Japanese authors. Thus Briedal [50] called this syndrome the "Japanese disease." Indeed, in 1960, Tsukimoto presented a case report with a post-mortem examination of a 47-year-old male with cervical myelopathy associated with a 3-mm thick intraspinal ossification posterior to C3/4. In 1964, Teramaya et al. reported a similar case and considered the compressing ossification to have developed within the posterior vertebral ligament, and to be neither arthrosis, nor ankylosing spondylarthritis, nor vertebral hyperostosis. In 1967, Onji et al. [259] reported 18 cases, two with biopsy: one of them was a haversian type ectopic bone. In Nagashima's 10 cases [253] all patients had been operated on. Operation revealed the presence of an osseous band in the anterior part of the spinal canal which was felt to be ossification of the posterior longitudinal ligament causing cord compression. Other cases have been reported: In Australia by Briedal [50], in the United States by Bakay et al. [16], and in France by Arlet et al. [10]. The latter surmised, however, whether his cases are not a matter of vertebral hyperostosis. Indeed, he analyzed 40 case reports of cervical myelopathy, and found 17 of them to have definite vertebral hyperostosis with (1) typical thoracic features, (2) no significant changes in the sacroiliac joints, and (3) acquired narrowing of the spinal canal by 9–11 mm of the actual anteroposterior diameter.

Our two cases are completely different and should be considered *dural ossifications* for the following reasons: (1) the anterior ossification is not only applied against the posterior aspect of the vertebral bodies, but also bridges the disks; (2) the posterior ossification lies at a slight distance from the posterior aspect of the spinal canal; and (3) finally, geometrical rules concerning roentgen projections favor a dural localization (see above).

C. Articular Fusion [177, 223, 310]

Synostoses are as rare as ossifications of the ligaments. Martel, Hohmann and Walcher, and Schilling et al. have reported on some cases. In most cases, it was a matter of bone ankylosis of the atlanto-odontoid articulation. Schilling [310] reported a case of irreducible atlantoaxial subluxation, which seemed to have bone tissue at the level of the enlarged articular interspace. One of our cases of psoriatic spondylarthritis appears definitely to show such an ossification (Fig. 72). This ossification process would correspond to repair or scarring, but we do not know if it is a specific process in ankylosing spondylarthritis.

As to the atlanto-occipital and atlantoaxial articulations, once they are destroyed by arthritis, they may undergo bone ankylosis. Contrariwise, we never encountered ankylosis which had not been preceded by arthritis. At this level, the evolution is identical to that occurring in the sacroiliac or in the zygapophyseal articulations.

D. Syndesmophytes and Hyperostosis

This type of lesion should be of frequent occurrence in ankylosing spondylarthritis. Such is, however, not the case. Pictures which have been described in detail in Part 5, Chapter 4, concerning rheumatoid arthritis, are exceptional here. Only Hohmann [176] reports arthrotic type changes in the atlanto-odontoid joint, without giving a precise description of the aspect of the bone constructions. Are they osteophytes, syndesmophytes, or hyperostoses? Hyperostosis, as we understand it, is located exclusively at the upper edge of the anterior articular facet of the odontoid process, and sometimes at the upper edge of the articular surface of the anterior arch of the atlas (Fig. 66). On frontal tomograms we found in four cases a "dens bicornus." We think that once more it is a matter of hyperostosis, the more the lateral edges of the odontoid are bordered by a linear opacity (Fig. 67).

E. Shining Odontoid

Under this term Martel [223] describes a reactive sclerosis of the odontoid, associated with erosion of the surface. Schilling believes this condition to be similar to that described by Romanus at the level of the lower spine and termed by him "anterior spondylitis" (Figs. 64, 66).

F. Hypertrophy of the Anterior Arch of the Atlas

The picture shown in Figure 68 may be interpreted differently. Is it simply a banal hyperostosis involving at once the cortex and the cancellous bone, or is it hypertrophy? According to Wackenheim [380], hypertrophy of the anterior arch of the atlas is almost necessarily associated with hypotrophy or even absence of the posterior arch, and vice versa. It represents a compensatory effect and is a frequent congenital anomaly without pathological significance. In the case reported the posterior arch of the atlas is poorly developed and it seems to be such a case of congenital malformation; we do not believe ankylosing spondylitis to be responsible for such images.

VI. Subluxations

All types of subluxations as we have described in rheumatoid arthritis are also seen in ankylosing spondylarthritis, i.e. transverse subluxation, rotation subluxation, atlantoaxial subluxation, upward luxation of the odontoid process, and forward atlanto-occipital subluxation.

The frequency of such lesions is not easy to determine since there are fewer series and cases published than in rheumatoid arthritis.

A. Anterior Atlantoaxial Subluxation

In all previous publications, only the atlantoaxial subluxations were counted.

Serre et al. [316] found 2 cases in 29 patients, Sharp and Purser [324] found 22 cases. These authors point out that the lesion is much less frequently observed in ankylosing spondylarthritis than in rheumatoid arthritis, but a definite prevalence rate could not be established from their study.

Schilling et al. [310] note that the cervical spine is clinically involved in more than half of the cases, and that radiological changes are present in 12% of the cases. According to this author, the rate of atlantoaxial subluxations would be of 2%. In a later study, he estimates the rate of atlantoaxial subluxations to vary from 2 to 8% in ankylosing spondylarthritis.

Finally, Hohmann and Walcher [177] made a roentgenographic study of 85 cases of ankylosing spondylarthritis, and found 10 atlantoaxial subluxations—a markedly higher percentage than is usually admitted. Among our 54 cases of ankylosing spondylarthritis in which X-rays of the neck were done, we found 3 cases with subluxation (Fig. 69), i.e., a percentage similar to Hohmann's. This rate is markedly lower than in rheumatoid arthritis (46% in our material).

Atlantoaxial subluxation has no specific features correlated with ankylosing spondylarthritis, and nothing distinguishes it from the same condition occurring in rheumatoid arthritis. Only the aspect of the lower cervical spine is different.

B. Upward Atlantoaxial Subluxation

This lesion has also been reported, e.g., by Hohmann, in some cases of ankylosing spondylarthritis. We ourselves never found such a lesion.

C. Atlantoaxial Rotation and Transverse Subluxation

In cases with arthritis of the atlantoaxial or atlanto-occipital joint, associated atlanto-odontoid rotatory and lateral subluxation can occur. These two subluxations are usually of minor degree, and can only be demonstrated by tomography.

D. Anterosuperior Subluxation of the Atlas [380]

We have found this lesion only in ankylosing spondylarthritis, viz. in 8 of our 54 cases (Fig. 70). Under normal anatomic conditions, the foramen magnum and atlas lie on almost parallel planes. In anteroposterior subluxations of the atlas, the anterior arch of the atlas is raised and the posterior arch is lowered. Bull's angle (or atlantopalatine angle) concerns the craniocaudal position of the atlas relative to the craniocaudal position of the hard palate. This angle is formed by a line representing the prolongation of the hard palate, and the line joining the midpoints of the anterior and posterior arches of the atlas. Wackenheim's evaluation of Bull's angle in 100 normal skull radiographs revealed values ranging from -2 to $+35°$ (mean value: $+20°$). The upper limit of normal is of about 30°, and only values of over 30° should be considered pathological. In anterosuperior subluxation of the atlas the angle is theoretically increased. In order to determine the length of the odontoid process, Wackenheim measures the distance between its tip and the level of the superior margin of the anterior arch. Normally, the odontoid tip lies at a level 1–2 mm higher than the anterior arch of the atlas.

X-rays of the neck in the neutral position revealed, in our cases of anterosuperior subluxations of the atlas, a mean value of 27° for Bull's angle (range 19°–38°); and the odontoid tip was shown to lie 3–5 mm below the level of the superior margin of the anterior arch of the atlas (mean value: 3.5 mm).

Though the measurements gave values at the limits of normal, the atlas is indisputably in an abnormal position, especially in the case illustrated in Figure 69, which clearly shows the anterior arch of the atlas to have lost its normal connections with the anterior articular surface of this vertebra. We believe this anterosuperior subluxation of the atlas to be due to hyperextension of the cervical spine, the latter being itself secondary to dorsal kyphosis. Note that in none of our cases their is neither "descent" of the odontoid process during flexion of the head nor exaggerated ascent during extension.

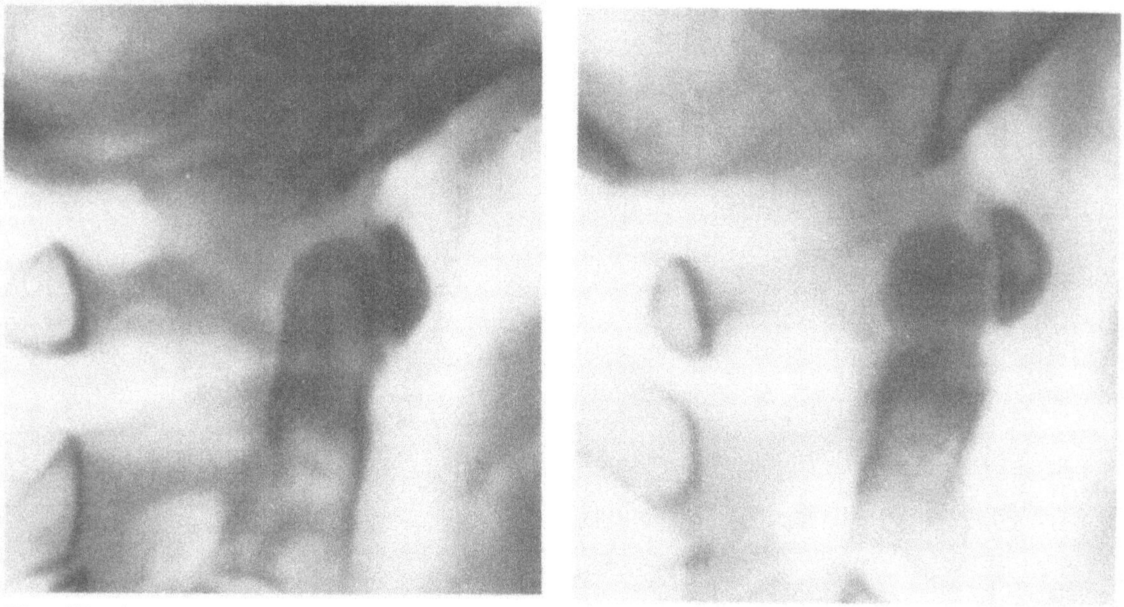

Fig. 70. Anterosuperior subluxation of the atlas in two cases of ankylosing spondylarthritis

E. Backward Subluxation of the Occiput

Without being specific, this condition is mainly seen in ankylosing spondylarthritis.

The first case with this type of subluxation was described by Coste et al. [80] in ankylosing spondylarthritis. According to Sharp and Purser [324], the involvement of the atlanto-occipital joints would be perhaps as frequent as that of the atlanto-odontoid, but the lesions of the ligaments of the former are much less frequent so that subluxations at this level are exceptional. Coste et al. wonder why an essentially ankylosing disease of little inflammatory type—at least as far as histological lesions of the cervical spine are concerned—may produce, in a quite sizeable number of cases, osteoarticular destructions causing subluxation in the cervico-occipital joint. The main factor is probably dorsal kyphosis with forward projection of the head and of the neck causing the upper segment of the cervical spine to carry the overhanging cranium.

VII. Radiofunctional Study of the Cervico-Occipital Joint

In this study we especially refer to the reports of Hohmann and Walcher [177] and to our personal experience.

The following questions may be asked:

May a specific evolution of the ankylosing process be seen at the level of the cervico-occipital joint? Is it possible to find hypermobility in the spared articulations?

Is there a correlation between progressive ankylosis of the cervical spine, and the occurrence of atlantoaxial subluxation?

The conclusions are interesting and may be summarized as follows:

In most of cases, ascending evolution of ankylosing spondylarthritis does not exist in the cervico-occipital joint. Even in

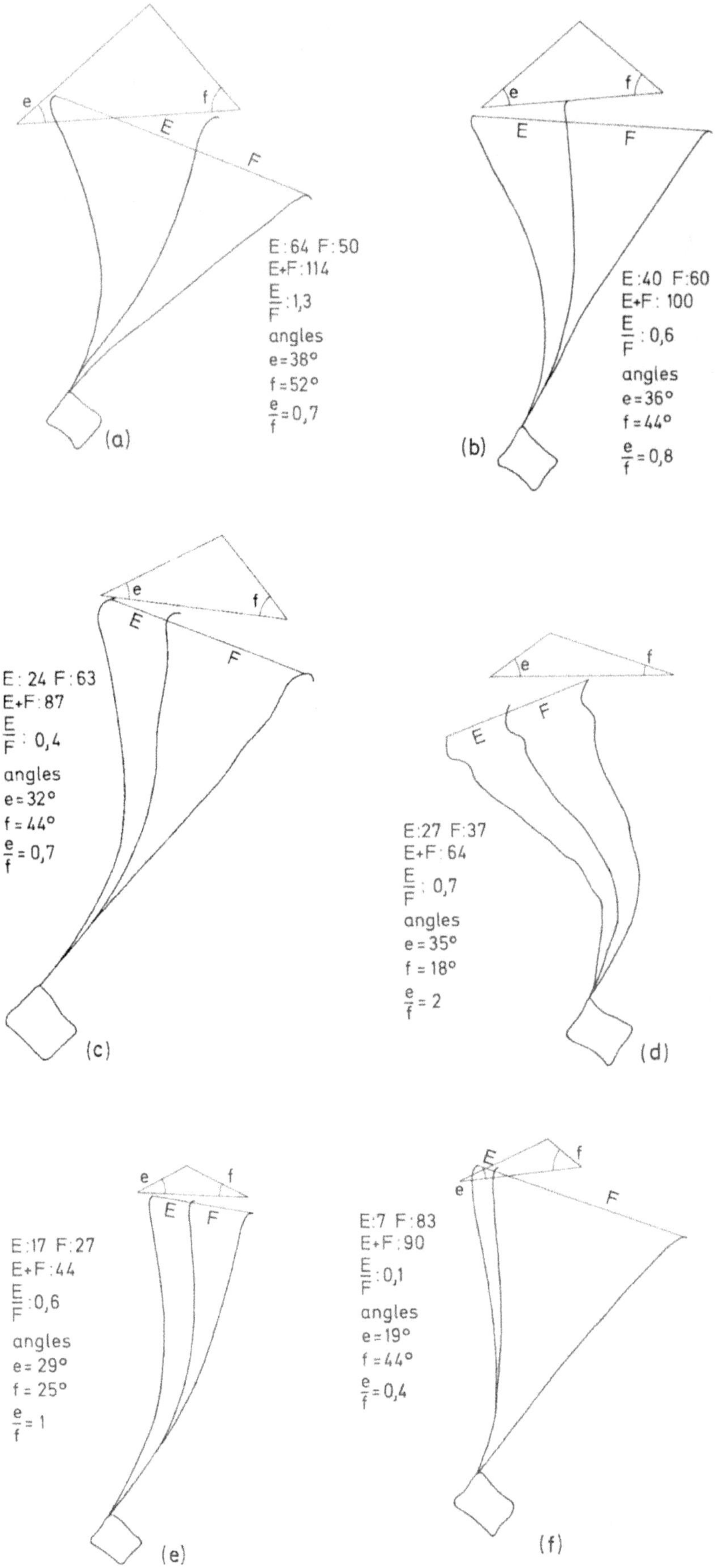
e
f
E
F
E:64 F:50
E+F:114
E/F:1,3
angles
e=38°
f=52°
e/f=0,7
(a)
e
f
E
F
E:40 F:60
E+F: 100
E/F: 0,6
angles
e=36°
f=44°
e/f=0,8
(b)
e
f
E
F
E: 24 F:63
E+F:87
E/F: 0,4
angles
e=32°
f=44°
e/f=0,7
(c)
e
f
E
F
E:27 F:37
E+F: 64
E/F: 0,7
angles
e=35°
f=18°
e/f=2
(d)
e
f
E
F
E:17 F:27
E+F:44
E/F:0,6
angles
e=29°
f=25°
e/f=1
(e)
E
f
e
F
E:7 F:83
E+F:90
E/F:0,1
angles
e=19°
f=44°
e/f=0,4
(f)

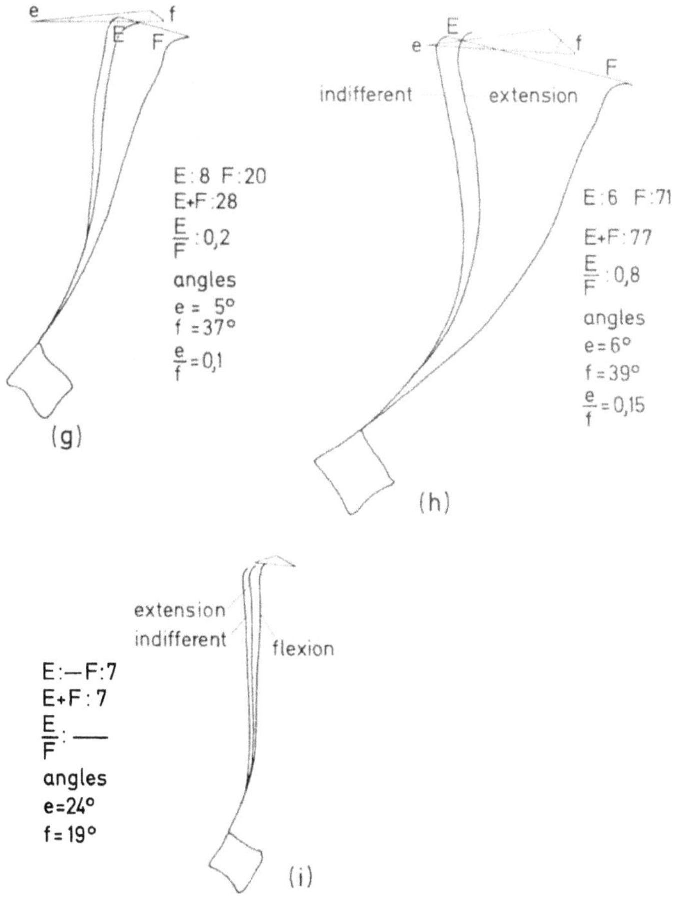

Fig. 71a–i. Wackenheim's method used for study of mobility of the cervico-occipital region and the lower cervical spine in nine cases of ankylosing spondylarthritis. **(a)** Hypermobility. **(b)** and **(c)** Moderate limitation of extension movement. **(d)** Hyperlordosis with relatively few functional disturbances. Note that this patient with non-reducible C1/2 dislocation has no "paradoxical extension" [see **(h)** and **(i)**]. **(e)**, **(f)** and **(g)** Predominant anomaly is the limitation of the amplitude of extension movement, without compensation of the cervico-occipital hinge. **(h)** and **(i)** "Paradoxical extension" characterized by a slight flexion between C2 and C7 in extension of the head. In both cases, there is a reducible atlantoaxial subluxation, i.e. hypermobility of the cervico-occipital hinge

cases with persistent mobility in the cervical spine there may be ankylosis of the atlanto-occipital articulations, whereas the atlantoaxial articulations are spared. According to Hohmann and Walcher, isolated involvement of the atlantoaxial articulation does not exist. Thus, the disease may spare certain joints and lose its strictly ascending character at the level of the cervico-occipital joint. The explanation for these findings would be the peculiar articular mechanics, as well as the special anatomic structure, but the above-cited authors do not provide precise arguments to support this hypothesis.

If there is progressive stiffening of the spine, the articulations of the cervico-occipital spine may, if they have been spared, compensate for the loss of mobility by being themselves more mobile. Indeed, Hohmann and Walcher found more atlantoaxial subluxations in those cases with stiffening or ankylosis of the cervical spine. Among their 10 cases with atlantoaxial subluxation,

7 had no mobility of the neck at all, and 2 had very reduced mobility. Our own findings are similar, i.e. on 3 subluxations, 2 had none while 1 had restricted mobility.

However, this does not mean that there is a direct correlation between these two conditions. As with polyarthritis, atlantoaxial subluxation would be due to involvement of the atlanto-odontoid and syndesmo-odontoid articulations. In practice, Wackenheim's cervical and cervico-occipital diagram (Fig. 4b) allows one to appreciate the evolution toward C2/7 stiffening with compensation at the level of the cervico-occipital joint (Fig. 71).

There exists a state in ankylosing spondylarthritis, where there is overall hypermobility of flexion and extension, of the C2/7 segment, and of the cervico-occipital joint. This hypermobility is related to lytic osseous and ligamentous lesions. Bony lysis may be very discrete (Fig. 71a).

The most frequently encountered functional disturbance is the limitation in C2/7 extension, compensated or not by relative hyperextension of the cervico-occipital joint (Fig. 71b–d). One may wonder to what extent the predominance of flexion and the resulting abnormal stress on the corresponding anatomical structures are responsible for selective destruction of the transverse ligament. In most cases, the condition evolves toward a more or less overall stiffening of the cervical spine.

In cases with fixed C1/2 dislocation (Fig. 71d) there exists hyperlordosis with relatively few functional disturbances.

A peculiar dynamic pattern – termed by us "paradoxical extension" – is characterized by the fact that the C2/7 segment carries out a slight flexion during extension of the head. Therefore, in the figure, the line of the posterior aspect of the vertebral bodies during extension is situated between the line of the posterior aspect of the vertebral bodies during flexion, and the corresponding line during the neutral position (Fig. 71h, i). These paradoxical dynamics are related to a C1/2 instability which results in C1/2 dislocation in flexion, reducible by extension.

The table below summarizes our findings based on 54 examinations in ankylosing spondylarthritis:

Rarefaction of bone	36
Atlanto-occipital arthritis	8
Atlantoaxial arthritis	3
Erosion of the odontoid process	14
Ossification of ligaments	3
Ossification of the meninges	2
Articular fusion	6
Syndesmophytes	0
Hyperostosis	8
Shining odontoid	2
Atlantoaxial subluxation	3
Upward atlantoaxial subluxation	0
Rotation subluxation	2
Lateral subluxation	1
Anteroposterior subluxation of the atlas	8
Backward subluxation of the occiput	0

Chapter 3 Psoriatic Arthropathy

Though psoriatic arthropathy has been known for a long time, its nosology is as yet not precisely demarcated. Indeed, several problems arise: When psoriasis and arthritis are present at the same time, is it always a matter of psoriatic arthritis? What are the connections between spondylarthritis in psoriatic patients and common ankylosing spondylarthritis?

Supposing that psoriasis predisposes to rheumatoid arthritis and modifies its biological, clinical, and anatomical features, that would account for psoriasis being more frequent in arthritic patients than in a random sample of the population, and for this deformed arthritis to be distinct from classical rheumatoid arthritis, thus producing the nosologic features of psoriatic arthropathy. The author does not believe that it is necessary to dissociate, as some do, the arthritides seen in psoriatic patients, or to differentiate a true psoriatic rheumatism from a rheumatoid polyarthritis associated by chance with psoriasis or from a mixed form, combining arthritis of the psoriatic type with rheumatoid arthritis.

This de-classification seems to be rather arbitrary, especially as concerns the mixed form. The first type, psoriatic rheumatism, seems to be by far the most common form. Epidemiologic studies grouping the HLA antigens would perhaps provide an answer to some of these questions. At the present time, eventual correlations between psoriatic arthritis and Reiter's syndrome are being considered. It is very likely that the search for urethral and articular inclusion bodies as well as immunologic tests, such as the lymphoblastic transformation test in the presence of Bedsonia antigen, would help to distinguish between these two similar conditions.

Finally, some authors [179, 192] have reported a certain number of osteoarticular changes in patients with psoriasis but free of any arthropathy. To give evidence of such lesions, these authors carried out systematic roentgenograms and scintigrams.

X-rays of the cervicocranial joint alone would certainly not provide the solution to the problem, but this examination might offer a new approach.

As with other inflammatory rheumatisms, there is also bone demineralization, arthritis, and different types of subluxations. Martel and Page [230] described one typical case of forward atlanto-occipital subluxation in psoriatic arthropathy:

"The anterior arch of the atlas had become reduced in thickness and the odontoid had also become small and pointed. These structures were displaced above McGregor's line but were considerably anterior to the foramen magnum, indicating that an atlanto-occipital subluxation had occurred. This was apparently followed by spontaneous atlanto-occipital fusion." Another patient with atypical spondylitis and mild psoriasis who developed an atlantoaxial subluxation was mentioned by Sharp and Purser [224]. Serre et al. [316] also report a case of a disabling polyarticular form of

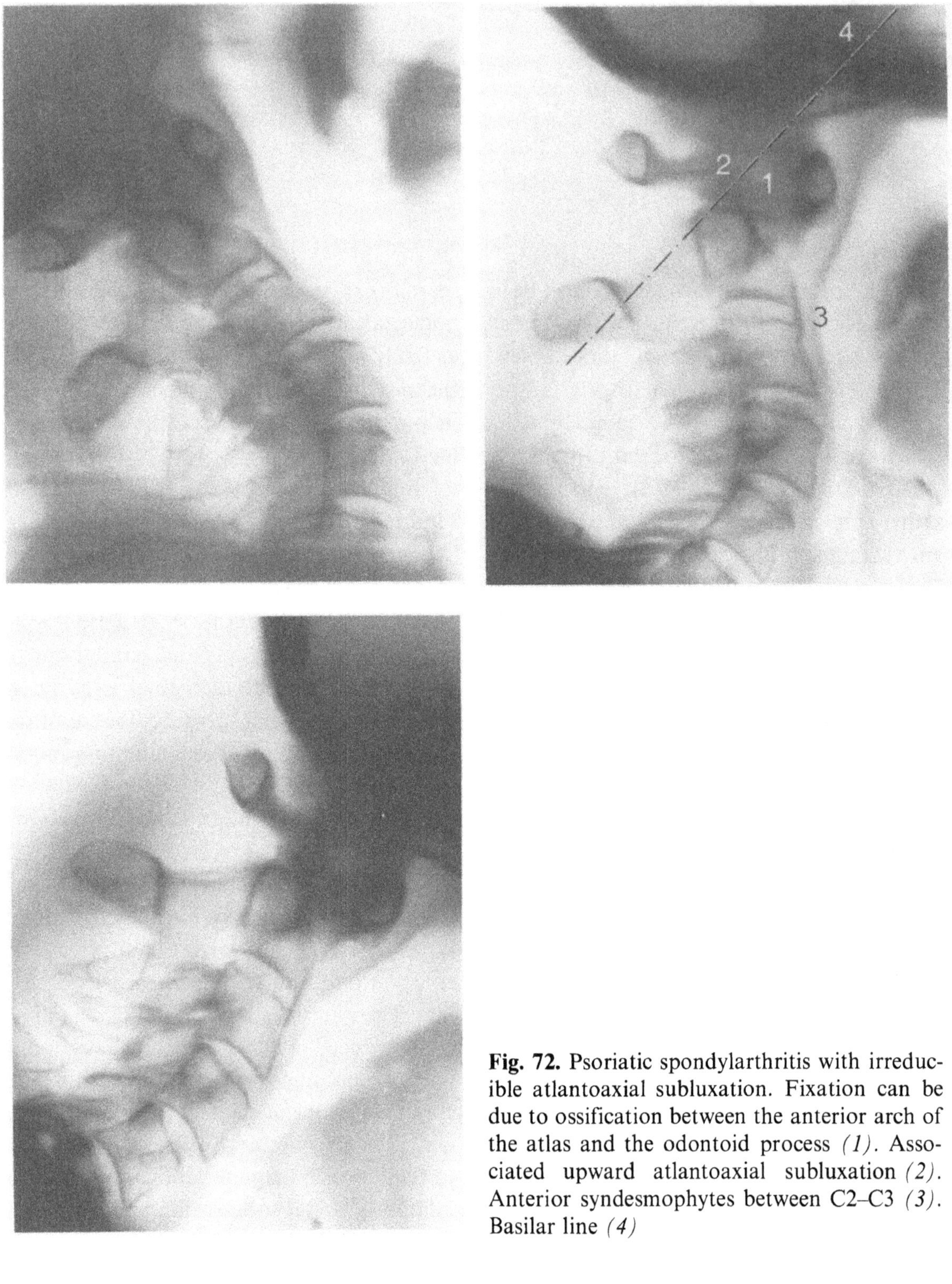

Fig. 72. Psoriatic spondylarthritis with irreducible atlantoaxial subluxation. Fixation can be due to ossification between the anterior arch of the atlas and the odontoid process *(1)*. Associated upward atlantoaxial subluxation *(2)*. Anterior syndesmophytes between C2–C3 *(3)*. Basilar line *(4)*

psoriatic rheumatism. This patient had signs of pyramidal tract involvement secondary to a 13 mm atlantoaxial subluxation. Four additional patients with psoriasis and roentgenologic evidence of systemic rheumatoid arthritis and abnormal atlantoaxial separation were mentioned by Peterson and Silbinger [274]. It is not clear if these patients also had spondylitis or distal interphalangeal joint involvement. Fi-

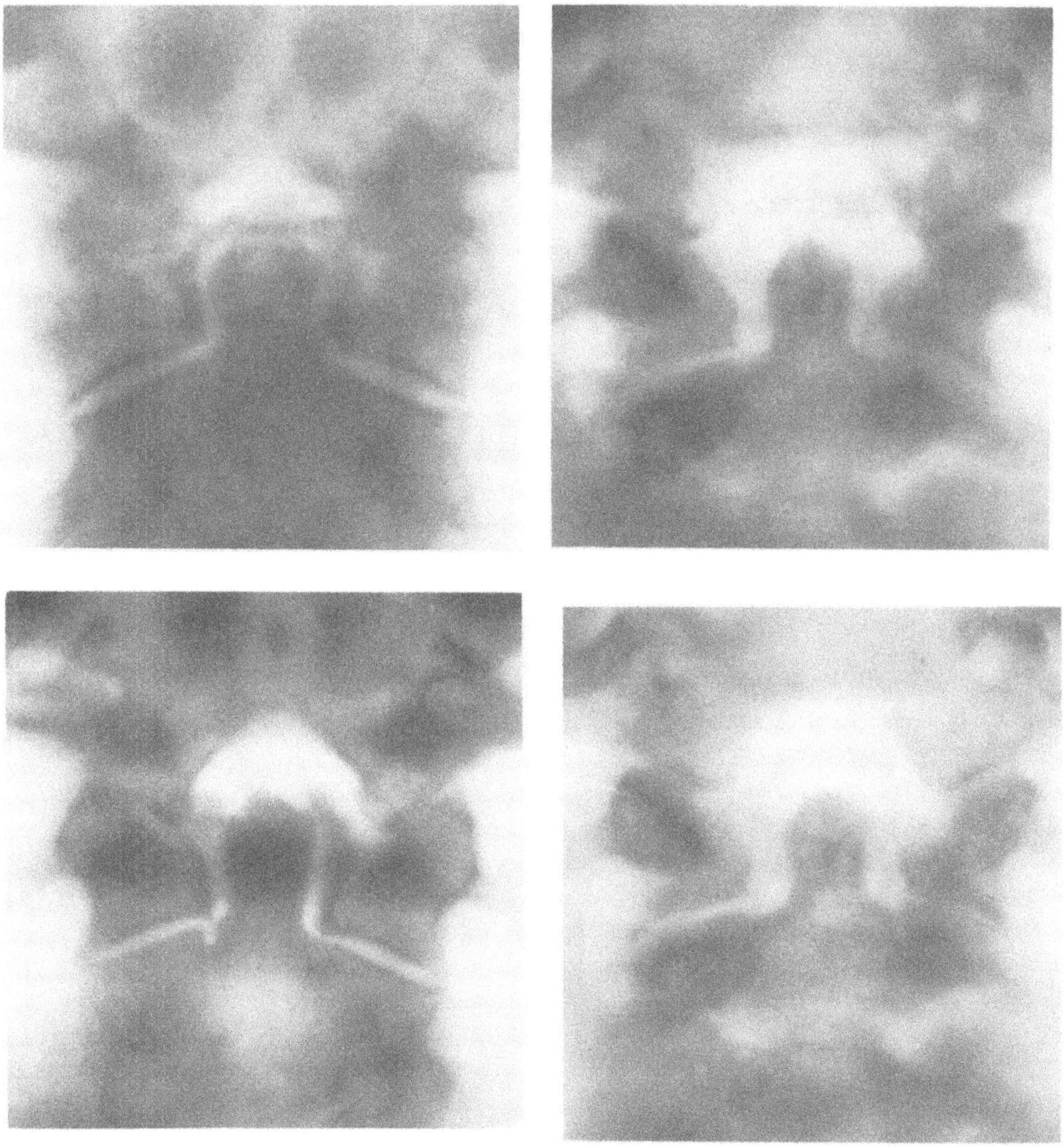

Fig. 73. "Crowned" odontoid in four cases of psoriatic arthritis

nally, Giuliano and Scully [141] reported a case of psoriatic arthropathy and atlantoaxial subluxation. The patient had neurologic symptoms consisting of several syncopal episodes and hyperreflexia of the lower extremities with sustained clonus bilaterally. A posterior fusion of the cervical vertebrae C1 through C3 was performed.

In our series of patients with psoriatic arthropathies, we found four *subluxations*: one case of simple atlantoaxial subluxation in psoriatic arthritis, two cases of upward atlantoaxial and anterior atlantoaxial subluxation in a case of psoriatic arthritis (see jacket cover), and one case of atlantoaxial subluxation in psoriatic ankylosing spondylitis (Fig. 72). There is no difference between these cases and those observed in rheumatoid arthritis.

The subluxations are by now well known. Contrariwise, *constructive bone lesions* have never been studied, though they

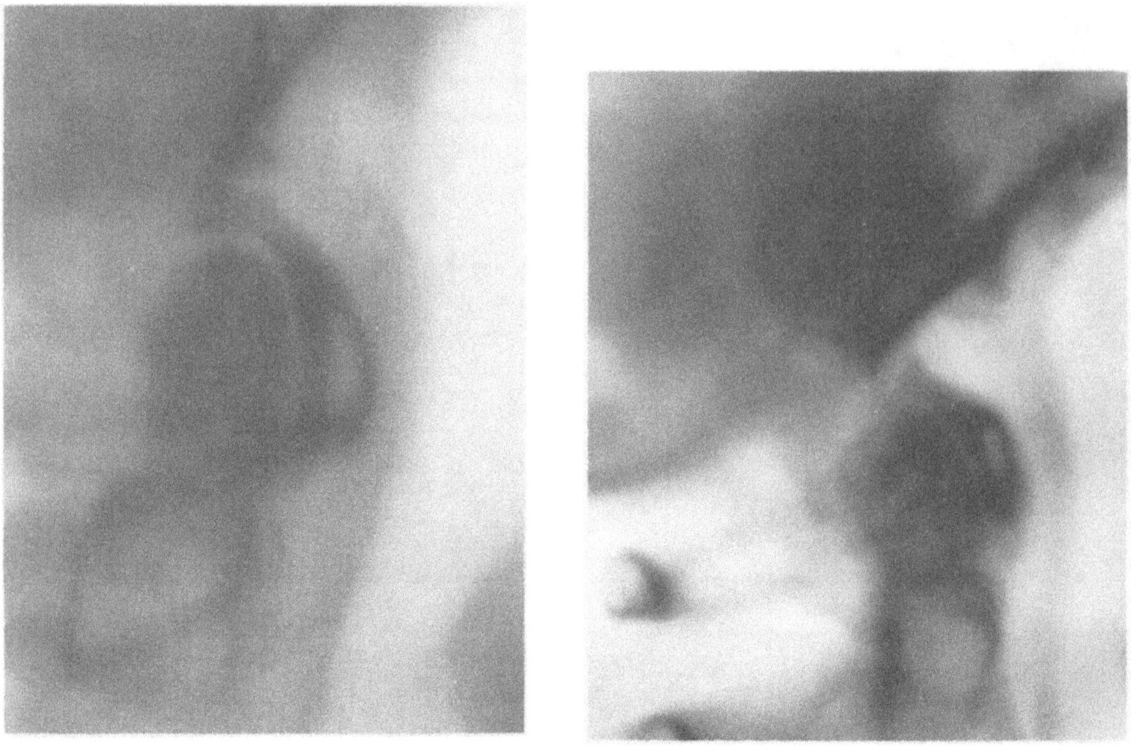

Fig. 74. Hyperostosis of the anterior arch of the atlas, and of the clivus in psoriatic arthritis

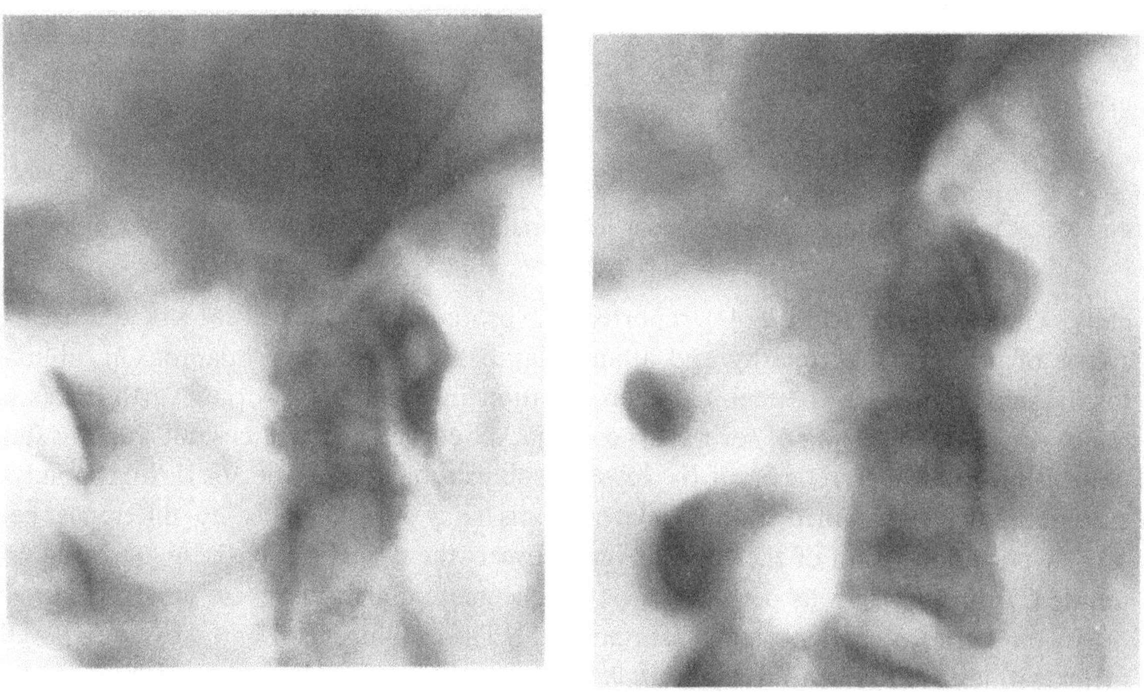

Fig. 75. Three cases of psoriatic arthritis with hyperostosis

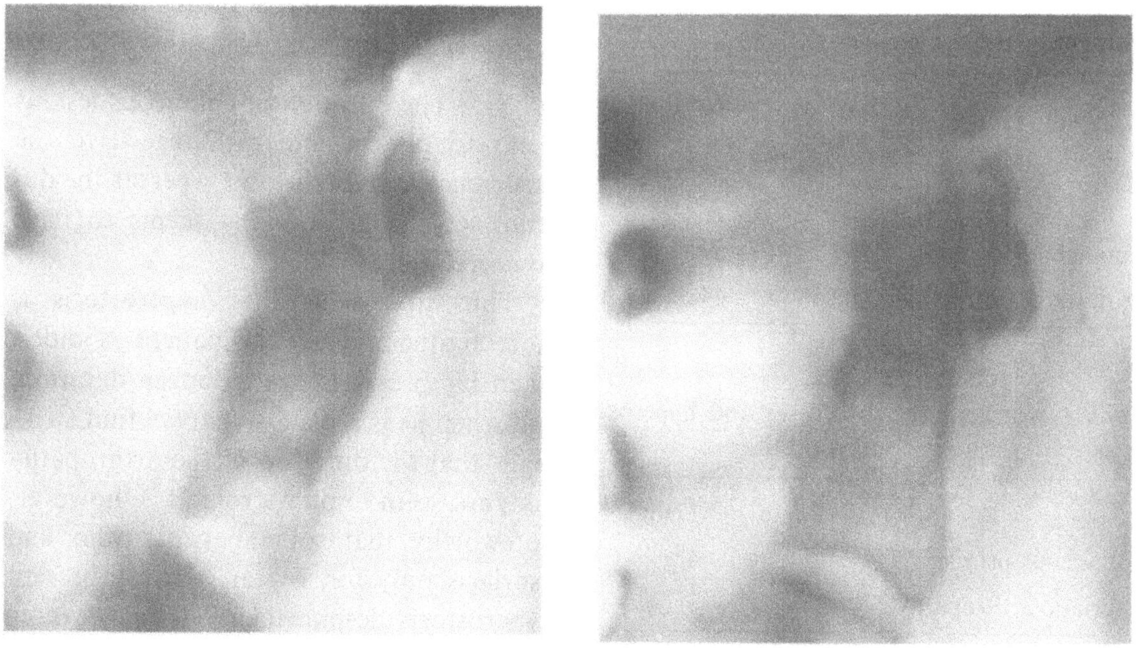

Fig. 76. Hyperostosis in two cases of cutaneous psoriasis without arthritis

are quite common (Figs. 73–75). Even Kaplan et al. [192] did not mention them in their study on the cervical spine in psoriasis and in psoriatic arthritis. Their radiological features have been dealt with in detail in the chapter on rheumatoid arthritis.

We would like to report the results of our own experience. We had the idea of comparing features seen in the cervico-occipital joint in patients with psoriatic arthropathy with those seen in patients with only cutaneous psoriasis (Fig. 76).

For this study, two groups of patients were taken, as follows:

1) Patients with seronegative psoriatic arthropathy: This group was subdivided as follows:

Psoriatic arthritis (18 cases), without sacroiliac or spinal involvement and without rheumatoid factor

Psoriatic ankylosing spondylarthritis (3 cases) characterized by the presence of uni- or bilateral sacroiliac arthritis associated or not with spinal syndesmophytes and with peripheral articular involvement

2) Patients with cutaneous psoriasis and free from any inflammatory articular involvement (16 cases).

Table 2. Materials

	Cutaneous psoriasis (16 cases)	Psoriatic arthropathy (21 cases)
Age:	22–74 Average: 51	27–78 Average: 55
Duration of psoriasis (years)	1–37 Average: 10	1–37 Average: 20
Duration of arthropathy (years)	–	1–25 Average: 10
Sex:	Male: 8 Female: 8	Male: 14 Female: 7
No. of patients with hyperostosis	9	14

Table 3. Comparison of average age of patients with and without hyperostosis

	With ossification (years)	Without ossification (years)
Cutaneous psoriasis	69	39
Psoriatic arthropathy	60.5	44.5

Table 4. Correlation between sex and hyperostosis

	Male	Female
Cutaneous psoriasis	5	4
Psoriatic arthropathy	7	7

Table 5. Duration of psoriasis (years)

	With ossification	Without ossification
Cutaneous psoriasis	13	9
Psoriatic arthropathy	20	16

In the group with seronegative psoriatic arthropathy the duration of arthropathy (in years) is 9.5 years in the cases with ossification and 11 years in the cases without ossification.

What conclusions can be drawn from these comparisons?

Table 2: The groups are similar with regard to average age. Distribution with regard to sex shows psoriatic arthropathy to be predominantly male—a classical notion. The dermatosis has a longer duration in the group with arthropathies than in the group with only cutaneous psoriasis.

Table 3: The patients with hyperostosis are older than those without, whether they have arthropathy or not.

Table 4: Sex does not seem to play a role in the occurrence of arthropathy.

Table 5: The duration of cutaneous lesions seems to play a role with regard to the occurrence of hyperostosis, whereas the duration of the arthropathy seems to have no correlation.

Thus, its seems that hyperostosis is more frequent when the patient is older, when his psoriasis has a longer duration, and when he is a male. What we find striking is that the duration of the arthropathy does not seem to play a role. It is, however, noteworthy that some patients who had psoriasis only for 1 year, already present hyperostosis despite their relatively young age.

As has already been pointed out, hyperostosis is also seen in rheumatoid arthritis, though less frequently. In ankylosing vertebral hyperostosis, the occurrence of ossification is the same as in psoriasis. Finally, in a random group of patients without rheumatologic lesions, such findings are very rare.

We did not take into account in these statistics the quantitative aspect of hyperostosis. However, it should be pointed out that the most marked and most advanced lesions are encountered in the group of patients presenting with psoriatic arthropathy.

What is the significance of hyperostosis? The different hypotheses have been discussed in the chapter on rheumatoid arthritis. As concerns psoriasis, the problem of the paravertebral ossifications described by Bywaters and Dixon [56] or parasyndesmophytes, as described by Dihlmann [98], also arises. The first authors had, in one of their cases, an opportunity to perform a postmortem examination. They noted that the new woven bone had a structure similar to periosteal new bone. They wondered whether this bone, apparently separated from the layer of periosteum covering the vertebral bodies, occurs at the site of muscle insertion into the paraspinal ligaments. One may wonder if the origin of what we call hyperostosis is not analogous to these paravertebral ossifications. (We would, however, like to recall that we have also seen hyperostosis in the craniocervical joint in rheumatoid arthritis.) Moreover, several patients have been X-rayed after a period of over 5 years, and there was no evidence of marked modifications of the hyperostosis. These findings are not consistent with those of Bywaters and Dixon who reported, in two of their cases, an extremely rapid evolution of the paraspinal ossifications, as well as of the periosteal ossifications involving the juxta-articular areas of the hands, feet, ankles, humeri, pelves, and femurs.

Chapter 4 Miscellaneous

I. Reiter's Syndrome

The original triad of Reiter's syndrome · urethritis, arthritis, and conjunctivitis – has been enlarged to include anomalies of the skin, the mucous membranes, the lungs, the cardiovascular and the nervous system. Several authors [232, 238, 274] have studied the numerous features which are common to Reiter's syndrome, ankylosing spondylitis, and psoriatic arthritis. Only slight clinical and radiological differences distinguish post-Reiterian ankylosing spondylarthritis from primary spondylarthritis and psoriatic spondylarthritis. In Reiter's syndrome the cervical spine can be affected alone or in combination with sacroiliitis; lumbar spondylitis usually precedes cervical spondylitis. The syndesmophytes may be symmetrical, marginal, and smooth – as in ankylosing spondylitis – or they may be characteristically asymmetrical, non-marginal, massive comma-shaped ossifications, attached or adjacent, but unattached, to the vertebral bodies, as in psoriatic arthritis.

The cervico-occipital joint, on the other hand, has been rarely investigated, so that, to the author's knowledge, only a few cases have been reported. Sharp and Purser [324] describe a case classified as "atypical spondylitis," since it was felt that the patient was possibly suffering from an incomplete form of Reiter's syndrome. Radiographs revealed forward subluxation of the atlas of moderate degree. The displacement was reduced by skull traction, and occipitocervical fusion was performed. Among our seven patients with Reiter's syndrome we had two with lesions in the cervico-occipital joint. In one case, it was a *posterior and anterior erosion of the odontoid process* which had developed in 6 months, the previous X-rays being normal. This lesion is similar to that seen in rheumatoid arthritis (Fig. 77). In the other case, it was a matter of *hyperostosing lesions* in the cervico-occipital joint (Fig. 78), primarily involving the anterior arch of the atlas, which is caudally prolonged by an ossified nucleus, whereas cranially there exists an important bony mass adherent to the anterior arch of the atlas. This is thick and strictly vertical and does not penetrate between the clivus and the tip of the odontoid. These two bone parts have a normal morphology. Frontal tomograms show the classical picture known as crowned odontoid [106]. When this hyperostosis is compared to that occurring in rheumatoid arthritis and psoriatic arthropathy, it is felt to be thicker, more irregular, and quite similar to that occurring at the level of the other spinal segments. In none of our seven cases of Reiter's syndrome did we observe atlantoaxial subluxation.

II. Connective Tissue Diseases

As concerns these diseases, we have, unfortunately, very few investigations of the cervico-occipital joint.

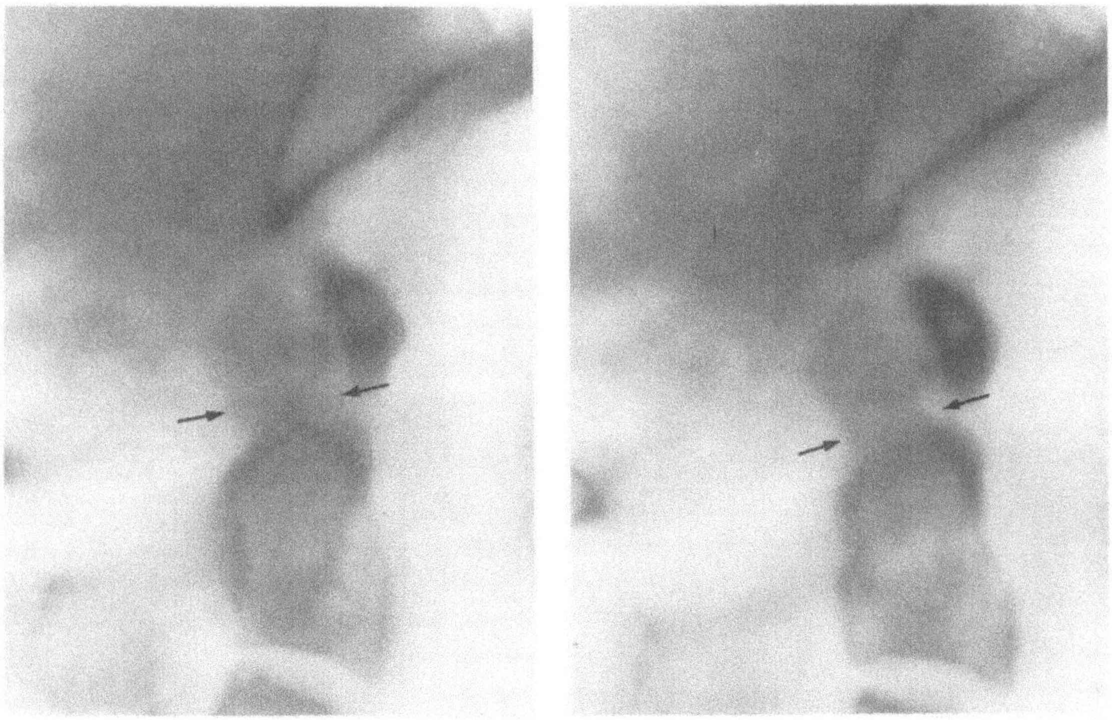

Fig. 77. Anterior and posterior erosion at the base of the odontoid process in one case of Reiter's syndrome. Six months earlier, X-rays did not show any abnormalities

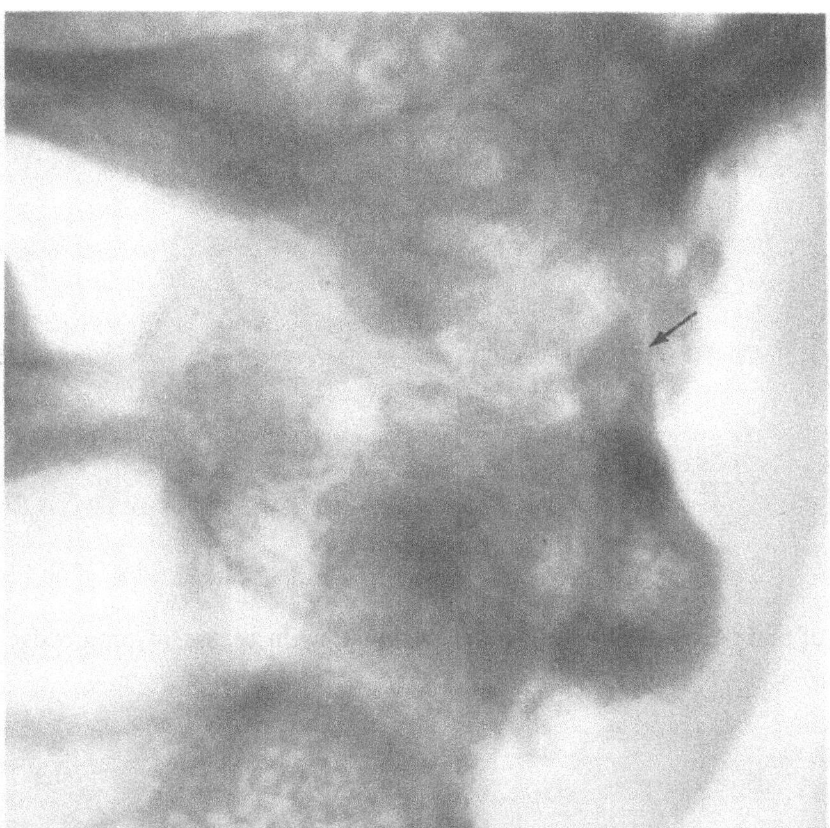

Fig. 78. Direct magnification in a case of hyperostosis of the anterior arch of the atlas in a case of Reiter's syndrome with onset 30 years previous

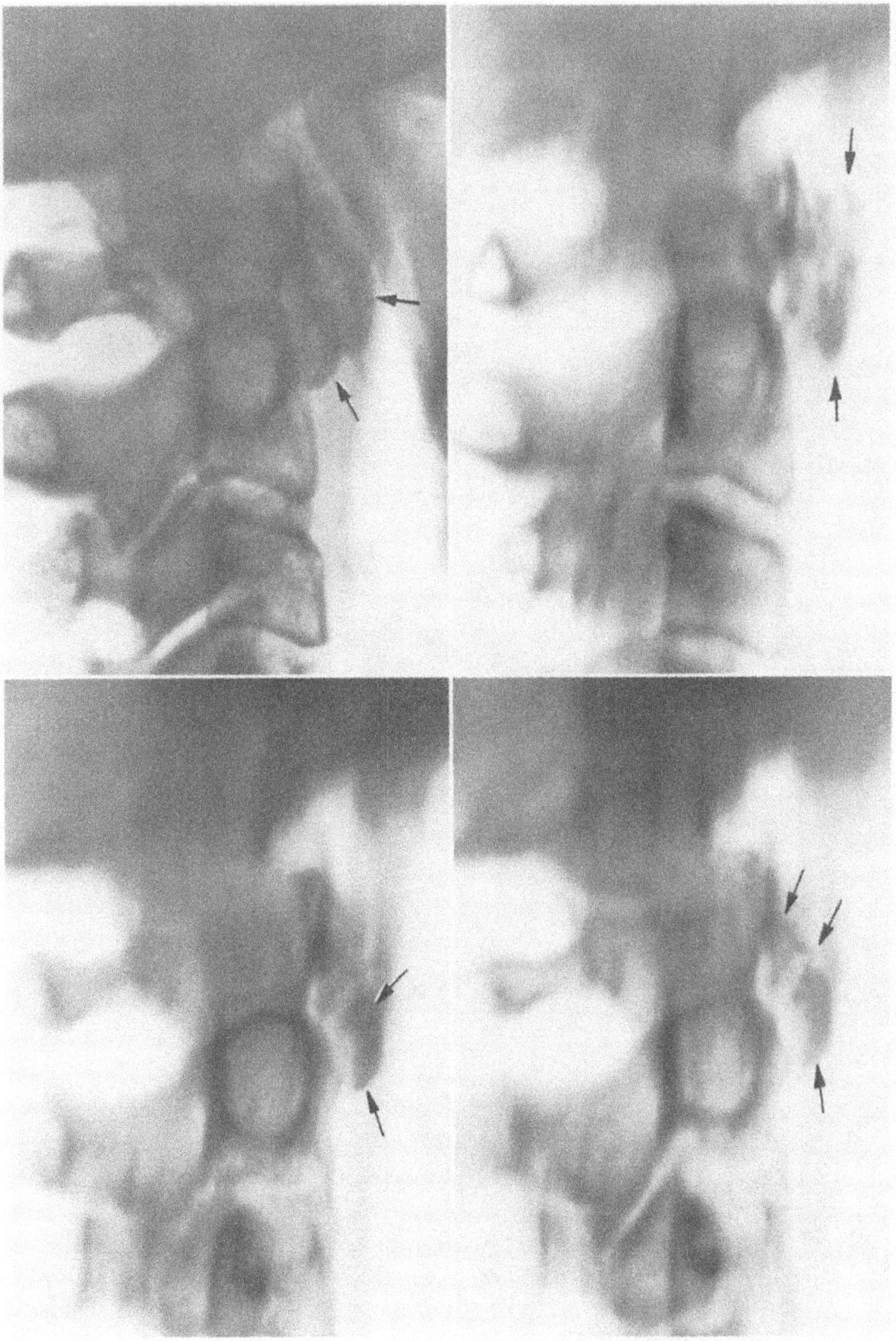

Fig. 79. Opacities in front of and below the posterior arch of the atlas in a case of progressive systemic sclerosis

A. Systemic Lupus Erythematosus

For this disease only Steinbach and Jensen [334] pointed out that X-rays may demonstrate subluxation in the cervical spine, particularly of the atlantoaxial joint. However, they cited no specific case in their own or other publications. Nor have we found any cases in our material or in the literature.

B. Progressive Systemic Sclerosis

In a case of scleroderma, we observed calcic or osseous accumulations in front of and above the anterior arch of the atlas (Fig. 79). It seems to us that if these were calcifications, their density would be higher. However, as far as one could judge, there was no bone structure. This condition is perhaps similar to soft tissue calcinosis, seen on the volar surface of the finger tips, and the metacarpophalangeal joint of the thumb, along tendon sheaths and bursae, described as the Thibierge-Weissenbach syndrome.

III. Behcet's Syndrome

We had the opportunity to examine the cervico-occipital joint in two patients with Behçet's syndrome and inflammatory-type chronic algia of the neck. Neither of these two cases showed radiological evidence of osteoarticular lesions.

IV. Intestinal Arthropathies

As long as a classification based on the etiopathogenesis is not available, certain syndromes and diseases are grouped either on the basis of current pathogenetic theories or with regard to clinical and developmental resemblences. Thus, we classify among the intestinal arthropathies, the arthritis in *ulcerative colitis,* in *regional enteritis,* and in *Whipple's disease.*

In these three conditions, chronic inflammatory rheumatism may be either arthritis or ankylosing spondylarthritis. To the author's knowledge, no cervico-occipital joint involvement has been reported and his eight cases had no roentgenologic evidence of such involvements.

V. Sarcoidosis

A complete radiotomographic study of the cervico-occipital joint has been carried out in a case of sarcoid chronic polyarthritis. Clinically, there was an inflammatory tenderness of the joint, but no X-ray changes could be seen.

Part 7 The Principles of Treatment in Lesions of the Cervico-Occipital Joint in Chronic Inflammatory Rheumatisms

In addition to the usual medical treatment of rheumatoid arthritis and other chronic inflammatory rheumatisms, the problem of a specific therapy must be considered in lesions of the cervico-occipital joint, usually subluxation. There are two choices: either conservative or surgical treatment.

In this chapter we shall deal with the methods which can be applied and the results, but will not describe the surgical techniques in detail. We conclude with the therapeutic indications.

I. Methods

A. Conservative Treatment

1. Abstention from Specific Therapy

This "non-medical" attitude is sometimes adopted with full knowledge of the case—despite the risk the patient may run—when the condition of the patient is felt to be too precarious. It should be pointed out that in elderly and bedridden patients the risk of a sudden accident is, nonetheless, quite lessened.

Also, in treating the arthritis, one would like to perform intra-articular injections or even synoviortheses of the articulations of the cervico-occipital joint. Unfortunately, no such technique is available; and even if synoviorthesis were possible, it would not solve the problem of the ligamentous lesions.

2. Analgesic Physiotherapy

Radar waves and ultrasound therapy have definite but mostly short-lived effects. Radiotherapy may also be applied; its beneficial effects in ankylosing arthritis are well known, whereas in rheumatoid arthritis the results are less consistent.

3. Massage, Physical Rehabilitation, Vertebral Manipulation

Since articular lesions are always accompanied by muscular contracture, cautiously performed massage may relieve pain temporarily in certain patients. We have already pointed out that any vertebral manipulation should be strictly proscribed and passive re-education avoided; as to active re-education, this will be restricted to simple exercises which do not induce pain.

4. Wearing of Minerva or Collar

Total immobilization in a Minerva cast or collar—when such is feasible—is not always well tolerated. In particular, there is a risk of cutaneous necrosis at the points of contact; besides, when fitted too tight at the level of the shoulders, e.g., in the case of ankylosis of the elbows, the patient may have some difficulty in carrying food to his mouth.

But often this device relieves cervico-occipital pains quickly and completely. Unfortunately, it is very difficult to convince a patient who suffers only moderately, and has no neurological symptoms, to wear such an apparatus.

All types of devices have been utilized: the Minerva plaster cast, the simple padded cardboard collar, the halo brace, plastic material padded with foam rubber, and moulded block leather. We ourselves have worked out a plastic Minerva cast allowing selective immobilization of flexion, extension, or both (Fig. 80). In atlantoaxial subluxation it is obviously the flexion movement which is to be suppressed, whereas extension is permitted.

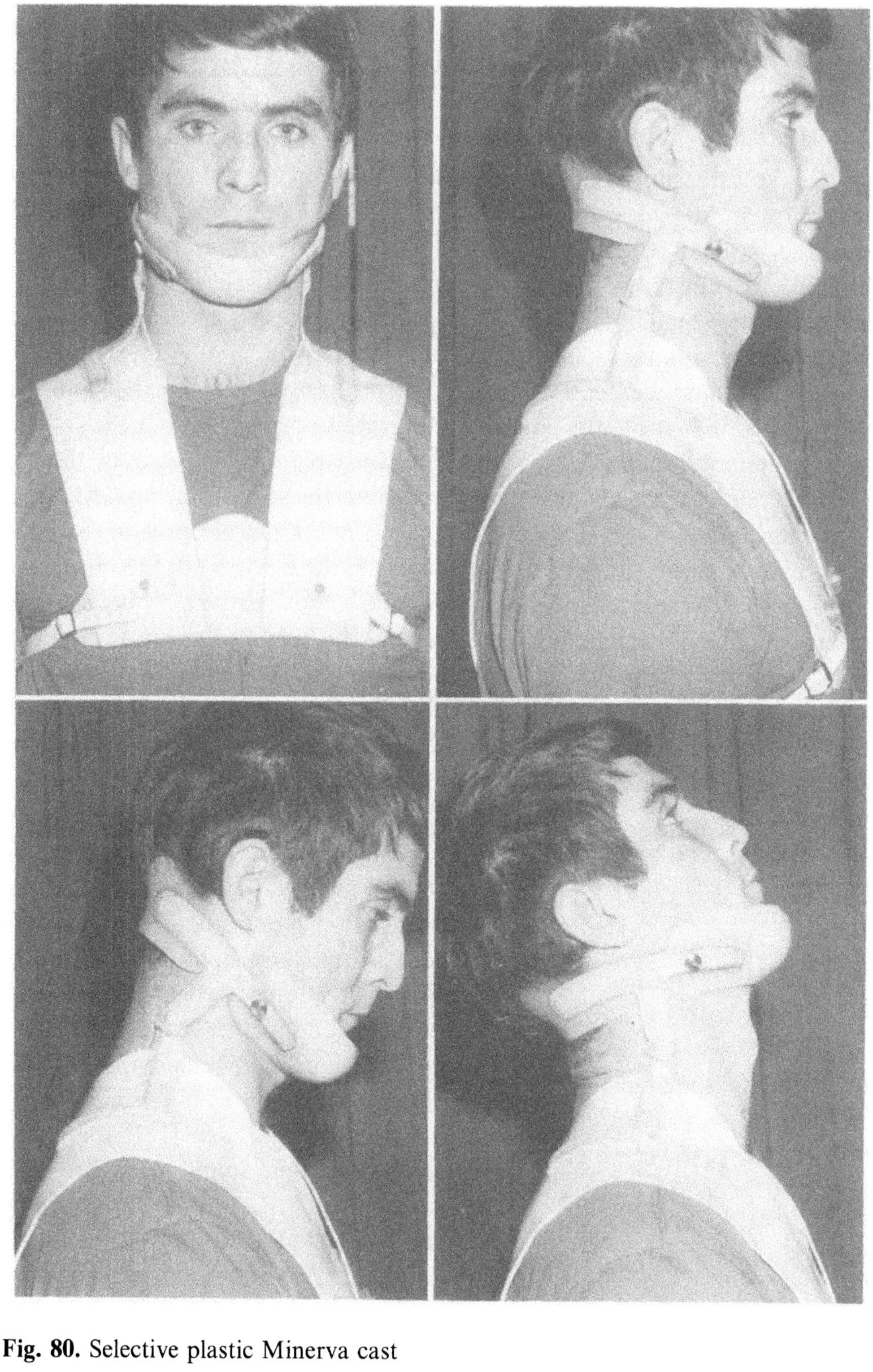

Fig. 80. Selective plastic Minerva cast

5. Continuous Extension of the Cervical Spine by Means of Cranial Calipers

The best procedure for trying to reduce subluxation by progressive extension consists in cranial traction by means of calipers brought to be on the parietal bones. This device is preferred to Glisson's sling. Crutchfield calipers or any model derived from this such as Blackburn hooks—may be used. The resulting continuous extension allows prolonged reduction but has to be completed either by immobilization by a collar or plaster Minerva cast or by surgical fixation. After the operation, continuous extension can also serve as means of clamping. The only drawback of these calipers is that they prevent the patient from getting up. To avoid this, some have thought of fixing the skeletal traction on a frame fitted into plaster. But this apparatus becomes heavy, cumbersome, and is not well tolerated by the patient.

B. Surgical Techniques

1. Decompressive Interventions

a) Laminectomy

Posterior opening of the spinal canal by resection of the laminae may be extended to several vertebrae, but is usually limited to the atlas. It can also be enlarged laterally by extending it as far as the lateral masses. It is possible to enlarge the foramen magnum upward by "resection of the dorsal margin of the occiput and opening of the dura, if traction proved not to give sufficient neurological improvement" [113].

b) Decompression by Anterior Approach

This is a more recent technique. Kao et al. [190] report a real *surgical synovectomy of the atlantodental articulation* through a transoral approach. It concerned a case of irreducible atlantoaxial subluxation in which the distance between the anterior arch of C1 and the anterior margin of the odontoid process was 15 mm. The operation showed that "there was tissue herniation above and below the anterior arch of C1 vertebra and the space between it and the odontoid process was densely packed with the same tissue. Four grams of this tissue were removed piecemeal under the dissecting microscope. After removal of the tissue between the anterior arch of the C1 vertebra and the odontoid process, and with the patient still under general anesthesia and under direct vision of the dissecting microscope, the patient's head was readjusted. Movement was seen at both the anterior arch of C1 vertebra and the odontoid process, and the distance between them was reduced to 4 mm." Thirty-seven days later "a posterior occipito-C1-C2-C3 vertebral fusion was carried out using 20-gauge wires and acrylic plastic reinforcement." The second method for transoral resection of the odontoid process is used chiefly for ascending subluxations of the odontoid, when the dens protrudes through the foramen magnum and further reduces the space for the spinal cord. The method used is a further development of the technique described by Fang and Ong [121] for metastatic diseases of the spine. It has been described by Sukoff et al. [346] and by Bratström et al. [47] for the treatment of rheumatic lesions of the cervico-occipital joint. The first reported case is described as follows: "the arch of the atlas was removed and a fusion of C2 to the occiput was performed ... Six weeks later, the neurological examination was normal ... Within six months the insidious onset of quadriparesis again began ... A cervical myelogram demonstrated an almost complete block at the foramen magnum ... A transoral removal of the odontoid process and rheumatoid tissue was performed." In the second reported case "the base of the odontoid process was separated from the body of the axis by means of an air-drill and the process was removed piecemeal. A small portion of the apex of the odontoid process, which was strongly adherent to the dura, was left in place ... After 3 weeks, a posterior fusion was done from the occipital bone to C2 and C3, using wire, pins, and acrylic plastic."

In all cases using the anterior transoral approach, it is necessary to perform, during a second intervention, arthrodesis by a posterior approach.

Only Robin de Andrade and Macnab [291] report a case of posterior decompression by laminectomy of C1 to C2 and where "an anterior cervical fusion extending from the occiput to C3 was performed ... Four slabs of cancellous autogenous iliac bone removed at the same operation were laid on the bare bone of the occiput and the C1 to C3 vertebrae. The anterior cervical muscles were allowed to fall back over the graft ... Examinations 6 years later revealed a painless neck with appropriate limitation of movement. Minor hoarseness of the voice had persisted. The plantar responses remained extensor, the tendon reflexes were normal, and pinprick and touch were normally felt. Joint position sense was normal. X-rays of the neck in flexion and extension showed fusion of the occipitocervical region."

2. Fusion of the Upper Cervical Spine

[6, 49, 63, 69, 82, 85, 91, 113, 146, 158, 211, 246, 268, 281, 285, 291, 295, 299, 357, 374, 398]

Immobilization of the cervico-occipital joint has been performed with numerous surgical techniques which are in fact only variants of a few basic ones. Two main types may be distinguished and preferred to others on account of the state of the joint, the data of the clinical and radiological examinations, and the functional results expected.

a) Posterior Fusion of C1 and C2 Vertebrae

This is theoretically the more simple of the two techniques. It consists in performing fusion of the posterior arches of the atlas and axis by a mixed arthrodesis combining graft and C1–C2 wiring.

In case of subluxation, one may try to reduce the displacement by pre- or peroperatory extension. The easiest way to obtain satisfactory reduction is to pass a loop under the posterior arch of C1. Both extremities of the wire are then knotted together under the spinous process of C2. Stability may be increased by screwing the graft.

b) Occipitovertebral Fusion

The graft is fixed under the external occipital tuberosity. A wire is passed around the posterior arch of C1 and knotted onto the graft. Finally, fixation of the graft on C2 may be achieved by simply embedment or, still better, by screwing into the spinous process of C2. In some cases, fusion may be extended onto C3. This technique has the advantage of allowing laminectomy or resection of the posterior arch of the atlas.

In this latter intervention and in order to increase stability, bone cement or osteosynthetis material is been used in addition to the wire.

These techniques have the great advantage of allowing the patients to walk around without a plaster Minerva cast soon, after the operation, whereas, normally immobilization is maintained until bone consolidation is attained, i.e. up to 3 months.

II. Results

A. Evolution in Case of Abstention from Specific Therapy

The result is the same as that of the natural evolution of atlantoaxial subluxation. According to Sharp and Purser [324] "... in 7 of the 9 rheumatoid patients given no specific treatment the displacement was producing no symptoms, and in one case it was causing minor pain. In one case the wearing of a collar was made impossible by an infection of the seventh cervical spinous process." None of these patients had neurological changes. In each of the six patients who had further radiographs 3 to 6 months after diagnosis, there had apparently been further narrowing of the canal.

Quite often we have abstained from specific treatment, particularly in patients in whom subluxation had been an accidental finding at X-ray, or in those who had no cervical pains. However, in 4 of the 38 patients in whom such decision had been taken, we recorded, over periods of from 5 months to 4 years, the occurrence of neurological symptoms – mostly minor but in one case major.

B. Results of Treatment with External Supports

Vignon et al. [371] have been using orthopedic immobilization in 14 patients of whom 6 had subluxations of 3–5 mm, and 5 of more than 8 mm. Five of these patients who had further radiographs over a year after diagnosis, showed persistance but not aggravation of the subluxation. These results are similar to those reported by Sharp and Purser [324] in a series of 13 patients wearing a plastic collar. These authors state that "to achieve virtually complete immobilization of the upper cervical spine by external means in an ambulant patient, fixation of the skull either by incorporation of skull calipers in a Minerva plaster or by a device such as the halo brace, is necessary." They go on to say that "X-rays taken in patients wearing a Minerva plaster showed that this external support does not immobilize the upper cervical spine and may not maintain reduction of an unstable atlantoaxial displacement. Any form of supporting collar which allows the patient to speak and to chew must also permit some upper cervical movement. Patients were therefore provided with supporting collars with the object of restricting cervical movement, relieving pain, and affording some mechanical protection from violent head movements. A not unimportant reason was that the collars also served to remind those looking after them of the presence of the lesion."

As for us, we use most often a simple padded plastic collar. By means of radiodynamic studies we could verify in several cases that the immobilization obtained is far from being complete, especially at the level of the cervico-occipital joint. Our plastic Minerva cast, with selective immobilization, renders the movements more limited, but it will not fully control subluxation.

We prescribed cervical immobilization in 18 cases. In a patient with atlantoaxial subluxation of 8 mm who suffered from unbearable left Arnold's neuralgia, pain could not be relieved and surgery was considered. In another case, the sensation of spinal instability disappeared but the pain could not be entirely alleviated. Since this patient had also rapid progressing erosion of the anterior arch of the atlas and of the odontoid (Figs. 13, 81), occipitocervical fusion was performed. In the 24 remaining cases pain has been practically relieved but there is evidence of aggravation of the subluxation in 4 of the 12 patients who had further X-rays within 7 to 32 months. In 8 patients the condition seems to be stabilized.

C. Results of Fixation Surgery

For this study we took the 13 most important and significant series to which we added 5 of our own cases (see Table 6).

1. Fatal Cases

In this condition, death is far from being a negligible eventuality since its frequency is 8.4%. This is due to two main reasons: either the neurological complications are marked and severe enough to entail death, or because death is inherent in any major surgical intervention. The risk is increased inasmuch as these patients are not only in poor physical condition but they are submitted to potentially harmful treatment such as corticotherapy, immunodepressive drugs, etc.

2. Unfavorable Results

These may be divided into two groups:

a) Failure of Fusion

This may be due to various factors—absence of fusion or lysis of the graft, rupture of the wiring, erosion, or rupture of the posterior arch of the atlas. To avoid such failure, double arthrodesis, i.e. simultaneous wiring and grafting, is now mostly performed. Also, to prevent rupture of the posterior arch of the atlas, occipitovertebral

Table 6

Authors	No. of surgical operations	Type of fusion		Results			
		C1-C2 (C3)	Cervico-occipital	Good	Fair	Bad	Exitus
Brattström and Granholm [49]	27		27	22	4	1	
Cregan [82]	6	3	3	4	1		1
Crellin et al. [83]	5	5		2	1		2
Creyssel et al. [85]	3	2	1	3			
Duyfjes [113]	14	?	?	9	2	2	1
Goutelle et al. [146]	6	4	2	5	1		
Hamblen [162]	5		5	2	1	2	
Ickovic [181]	6		6	2	1		3
Meyers et al. [246]	11	1	10	8	2		1
Robinson [292]	3		3	3			
Sharp and Purser [324]	4		4	3			1
Sweetnam [348]	9		9	9			
Thomas [357]	15	?	?	10	1	3	1
Personal cases	5	3	2	2	2	1	
Total	119	18	72	84	16	9	10
Percentage		20	80	70.6	13.4	7.6	8.4

arthrodesis is prefered to C1–C2 fusion. Since the posterior arch of the atlas is often hypoplastic and highly demineralized, fusion of the graft is not easily obtained, and postoperatory immobilization is often not properly achieved. We have also seen resorption of the graft in three interventions on two patients, both having been treated over a long time with prednisolone. The first of these two cases was described in the chapter on the influence of trauma on atlantoaxial subluxation. The second patient (Figs. 83–86), who presented a symptomatology of vertebrobasilar insufficiency, had a C1/C2 fusion performed. Six weeks after the operation and wearing a plastic Minerva cast which does, however, not immobilize him completely, he experiences marked vertigo on the occasion of brisk movement. X-rays of the neck disclose lysis of the graft at the level of the posterior arch of the axis. In addition, the atlantoaxial subluxation that had been reduced is again present though less marked than before the operation. A new intervention was done and a C0/C1/C2 fusion performed, but this, unfortunately, has failed to reduce the diastasis entirely. After a 3 months' immobilization, the graft is resorbed at the level of its occipital insertion and the atlantoaxial subluxation is partly mobile; the neurological symptoms, however, have disappeared.

Thus, it would seem that incomplete reduction of the atlantoaxial subluxation is not an unfavorable result: what counts is the maintenance of the function.

We have already partly quoted the very instructive case published by Sukoff et al. According to these authors "the initial results of removal of the arch of the atlas and posterior fusion were gratifying in our case. However, six months postoperatively, progressive myelopathy again developed despite evidence of occipitoatlantal stability on plain films. Myelography demonstrated a subtotal block suggesting anterior compression from a progressive posterior displacement of the dens. In this instance only the anterior approach was possible for decompression ... The patient made a total neurological recovery."

b) Poor Functional Results

Very exceptionally, cervico-occipital pains do not subside after arthrodesis. Persistence of neurological signs, their incomplete regression, or their recurrence have been pointed out by 8 of the 12 authors cited. Contrary to the opinion of Sweetnam, it is not always abstention from laminectomy which is the cause of failure. The report of Sukoff et al. is significant from this point of view. It raises the problem of indication of preoperative myelography. As we stated in Part 5, Chapter 6, we think that myelography is indicated in very specific cases.

Another cause of failure is when intervention is not done early enough, so that neurological manifestations persist indefinitely as in spondylitic myelopathy.

3. Reduction of Cervical Mobility Due to Fusion

Any fusion reduces mobility. As concerns the cervico-occipital hinge, a review of the physiology shows that it is a complex articular structure, and that sometimes some mobility may persist.

Occipitovertebral fusion blocks the atlantoaxial articulations and diminishes rotation by 40°. The remaining 45° will induce in the last five cervical vertebrae a lateroflexion on the side of the rotation due to the obliquity of the posterior articular processes. Moreover, pure lateroflexion is lost due to suppression of the antirotation movements of the atlas. It will thus thereafter combine with a rotation movement on the same side. Finally, the blocked occipitoatlantal articulation makes the spine lose 15° in flexion-extension. These 15° added to the loss of 15° flexion-extension allowed by the atlantoaxoid articulation entail a global loss of 30° of movements in the sagittal plane after arthrodesis.

C1/C2 arthrodesis produces a diminution of 40° of atlantoaxial rotation, and only of 15° of flexion-extension. Finally, C1/2/3 arthrodeses have the advantage, as do the previous ones, of keeping the atlanto-occipital articulation free. But they enable important blocking of three cervical segments and influence flexion-extension and lateroflexion.

In conclusion, it can be said that rotation is the movement which is most impeded by such interventions. Theoretically, it is supressed, but we came across case reports mentioning the persistence of some rotation (Rose [295]; Patte [268]; Sweetnam [348]), especially in patients under 40. Lateroflexion of small amplitude in the occipitoatlantal articulation may be maintained by cervical fusion. Contrariwise, it is suppressed in cervico-occipital fusion.

As to the flexion-extension movement, it is usually conserved to a satisfying degree in these three types of intervention. Besides, it seems that the reduction in mobility bears especially on extension.

Functional impairment secondary to such interventions is usually well tolerated by the patients. It goes without saying that since arthrodeses bring about functional overexertion of the lower cervical spine, the state of the latter should be examined before operation and taken into account in the choice of intervention.

4. Influence of Cervico-Occipital Fusion on the Lower Cervical Spine

We would like to quote Boyle [45] who thinks "the operation of occipitocervical fusion, so ably described by Newmann and Sweetnam [257] as 'a safe, simple, and above all reliable method' of stabilizing the atlantoaxial joint, certainly seems on the surface to be the operation of choice at the present time. Moreover, we know from experience that total fixation of other parts of the spine is not infrequently followed by lesions above or below the immobile segment. Because of this, we have for some time been concerned that total fixation of the upper cervical spine might lead to increasing strain and hence increasing instability due to rheumatoid arthritis happened already to be present. The following case may well be an illustration of such an event; Mrs. W.H. developed classical rheumatoid arthritis at the age of 52. Eleven years later, she experienced upper cervical pain and occipital headaches, difficulty in walking, and paresthesiae in the feet. Examination showed a spastic tetraparesis, and X-rays of the cervical spine revealed an atlantoaxial subluxation in flexion of 8 mm with disk narrowing, but no subluxation at C3/4 and C4/5 levels. Myelography showed no obstruction below C2. An occipitocervical fusion was successfully carried out and was followed by a rapid improvement in the tetraparesis to the extent that she was able to lead an almost normal life. Six months later she suddenly developed flexor spasms in the legs and hyperesthesia in all four limbs and became unable to walk. Examination showed a Brown-Sequard syndrome with impairment of sensation up to C5 level, with severe pyramidal signs in all four limbs. Further X-rays showed the atlantoaxial joint to be entirely stable, but a major slip of 5 mm had now occurred at C3/4 and a lesser slip at C4/5. The patient died within a few days from progressive cord involvement. Autopsy confirmed the subluxation at C3/4 and C4/5 where severe cord compression had occurred." We have not found another similar case in the literature. As concerns our four patients who are regularly followed-up clinically as well as radiologically, no changes in the lower cervical spine were recorded, not even in the case illustrated in Figure 84, which shows major multilevel spondylitis. Systematic follow-up examinations are indispensable once a year.

To prevent such complications, we recommend in case of diastasis with C2/3 kyphosis in flexion (Figs. 42, 43), incorporation of the C2/3 space into the arthrodesis, though we favor as small as possible an arthrodesis.

III. Therapeutic Indications

As soon as there is evidence of atlantoaxial subluxation, the therapeutic indications should be carefully considered and periodically discussed with regard to the evolution. They depend on numerous factors and especially on:

The age of the patient and his functional capacity

The general status and condition of the articulations, as well as the evolution of the arthritis

The degree of subluxation and its eventual evolution, and subsequent symptoms

The evolution of the neurological manifestations

The lesions which may be associated.

A. Indications for Conservative Treatment

Conservative treatment is conceivable in some circumstances. It is first applied in previously latent atlantoaxial subluxations—either spontaneous or provoked by flexion, or fixed or reducible by extension. These subluxations must, however, be of some extent. As we have already pointed out, as a measurement of the diastasis we prefer to compare the anteroposterior diameter of the vertebral canal of the atlas with the anteroposterior diameter of the vertebral canal of the axis. This method gives a better picture of the effect of the bone displacement on the medulla oblongata. Patients in whom measurements show these two diameters to be equal wear a Minerva cast. In the case of cervical pains related to the diastasis, it is necessary first to try all the medical and physiotherapeutic means we have quoted. When these fail to improve the condition, we use a clamping device which often gives satisfactory results. In addition, some patients complain of a sensation of instability of the head, an impression of dismantling of the head following certain movements, or of perception of a crepitus, which may even be heard by the examiner. These patients readily consent to wearing a clamping device. Moreover, the patients with a cervical myelopathy of cervico-occipital origin or a vertebral artery insufficiency, or those in whom a generally bad condition does not allow operation, must also be provided with such an apparatus. If, however, operation is contraindicated because of cardiac or respiratory insufficiency, wearing a clamping device, in particular a Minerva plaster cast, will not be well tolerated. The patients may sometimes benefit from skull traction which results in regression of neurological symptoms and, sometimes even, reduces the sub-

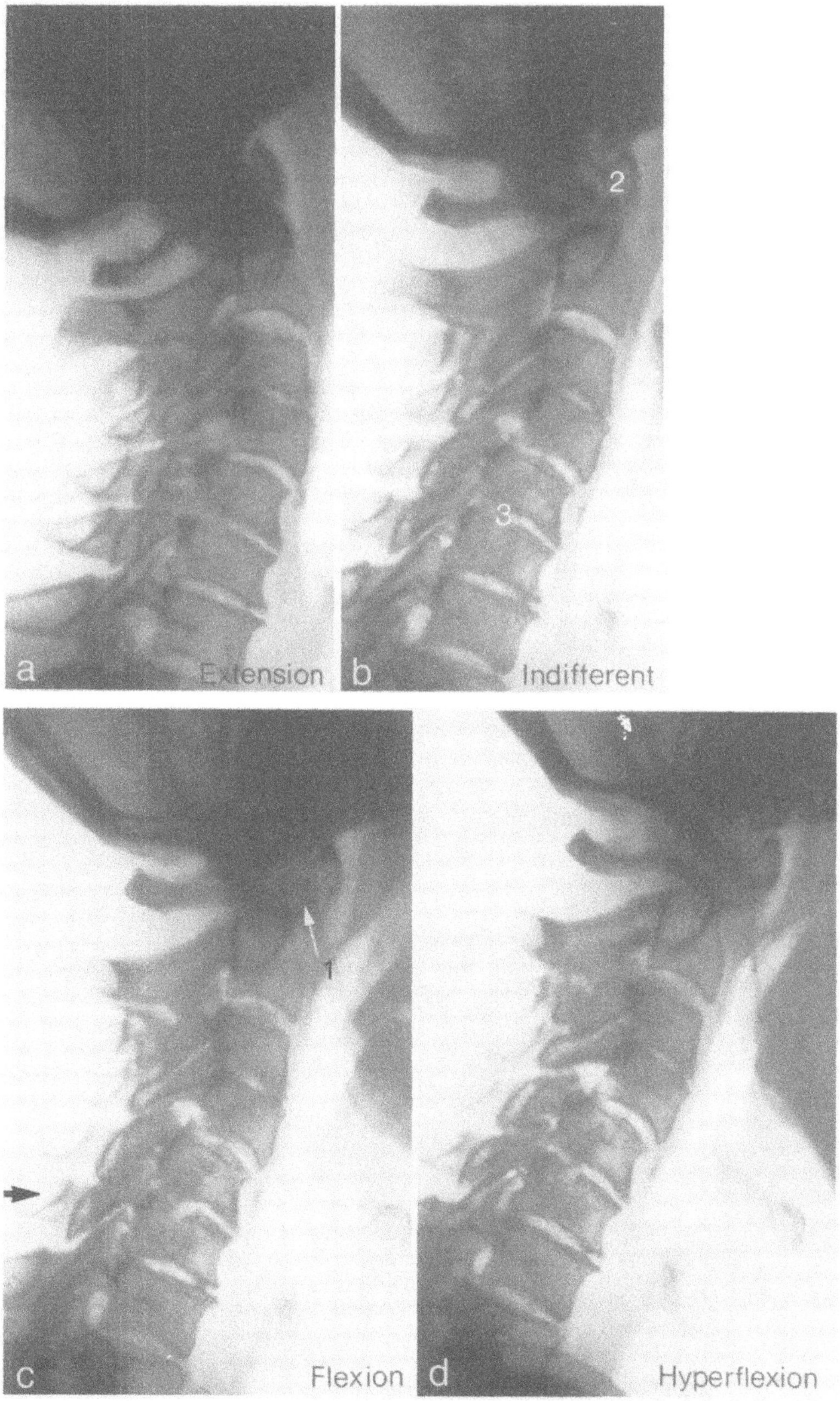

Fig. 81. Sensation of instability and crepitus between **(b)** and **(c)** position *(arrow)*, i.e., between the neutral and slightly flexed position (crepitus was audible by the examiner). (See also Fig. 83.) *1* Reducible C1/2 diastasis, *2* Erosion of posterior aspect of the anterior arch of the atlas, *3* Multiple spondylodiscitis

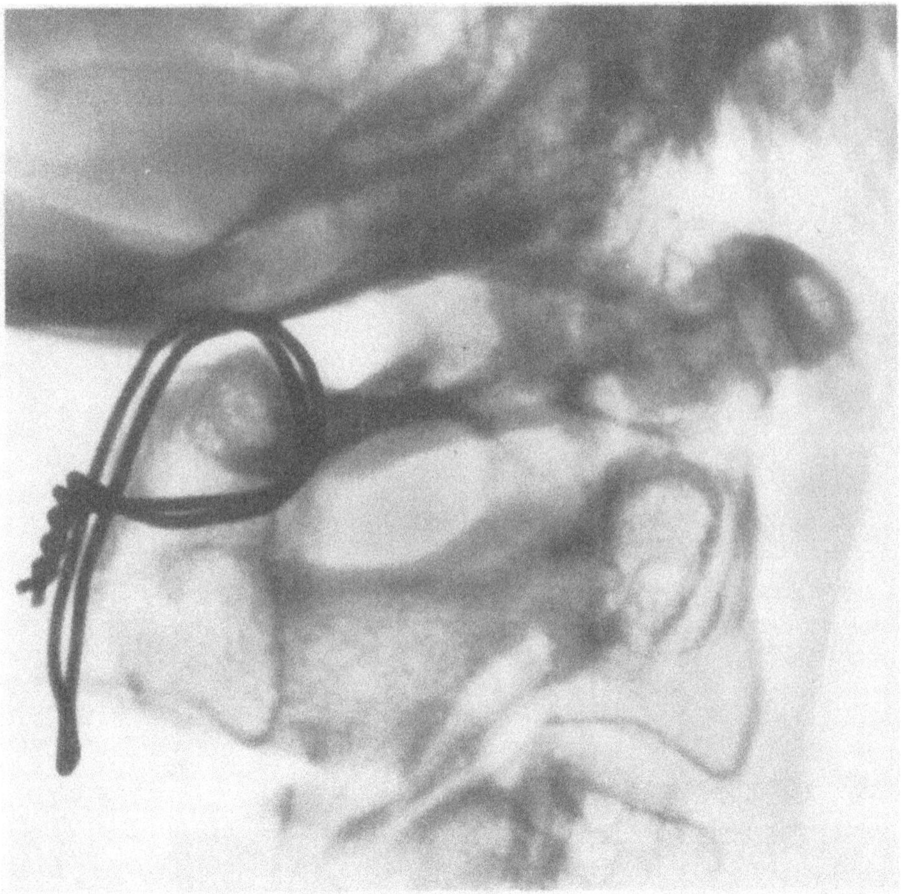

Fig. 82. Graft and wire for C1/2 fusion in a case of atlantoaxial diastasis in rheumatoid arthritis with satisfying results

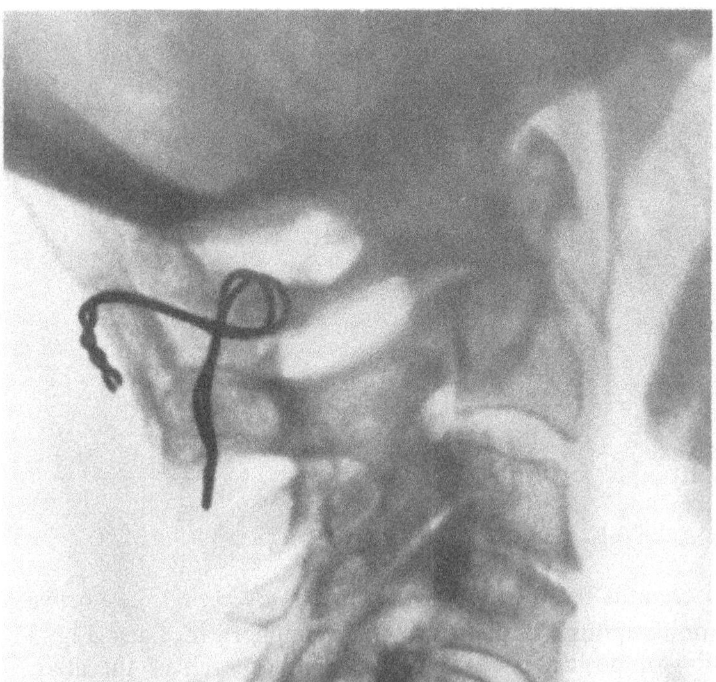

Fig. 83. In this patient, as illustrated in Fig. 81, a C0/C1/C2 fusion was performed with satisfactory results

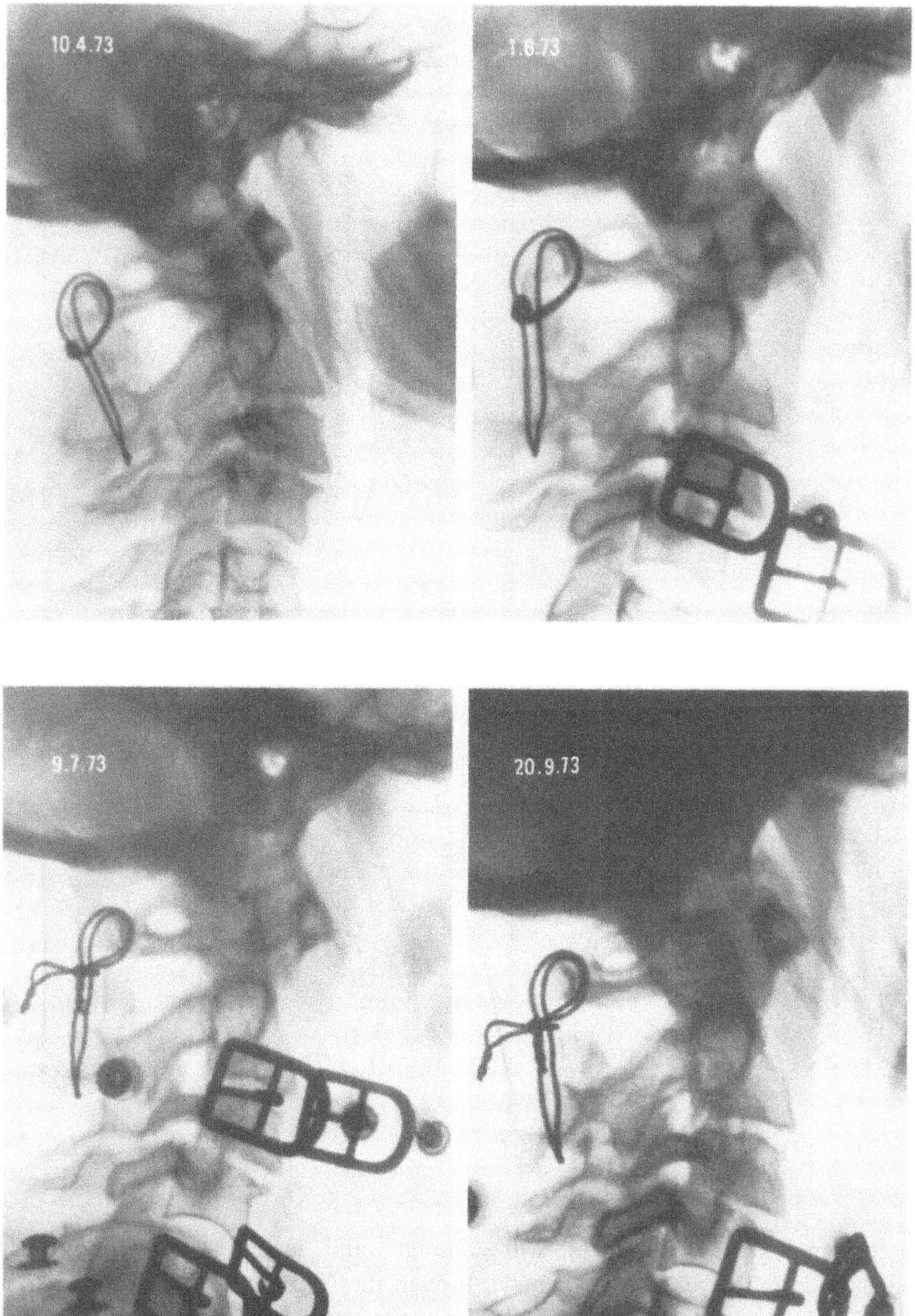

a

b

c

Fig. 84a–c. Unsuccessful operations in a case of rheumatoid arthritis. Preoperative examinations: see Fig. 36. Note that the diastasis is reducible in extension. Postoperative examinations: **(a)** After the first operation (fusion C1/2): 10.4.73 (1 week after operation) and 1.6.73: note that graft, still visible at the first control (10.4.73) is detached from the axis and is less opaque (1.6.73). (See Fig. 85.) **(b)** After second operation (fusion C0/C1/C2) one observes the same evolution i.e. the graft is visible on 9.7.73 (1 week after operation), is resorbed on the X-ray control of 9.7.73. The diastasis is incompletely reduced. **(c)** Eleven months after the second operation both grafts have practically disappeared (Fig. 86)

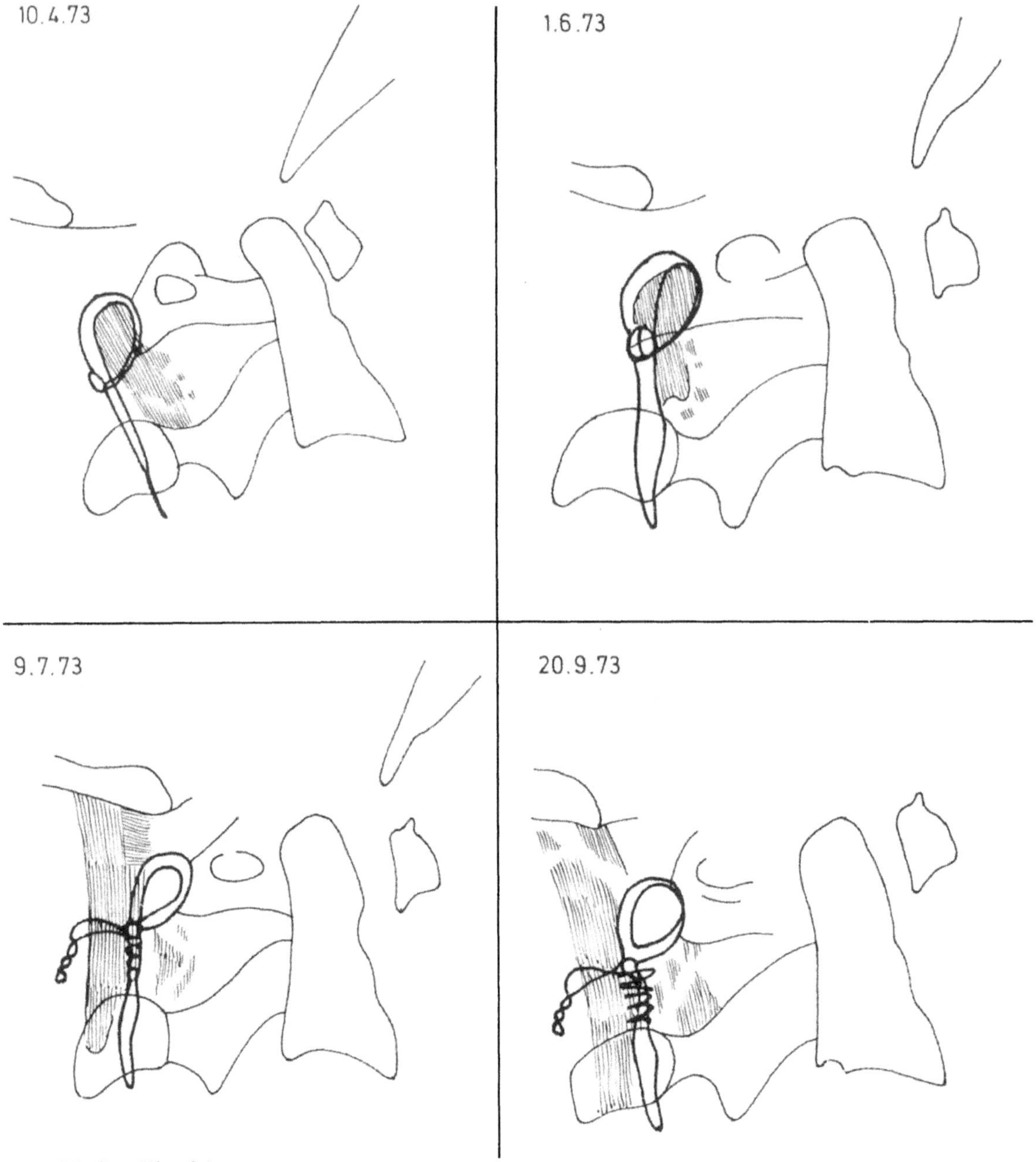

Fig. 85. See Fig. 84

luxation to some extent. Later on, it will be possible to immobilize these patients' cervical spine by means of an external clamping device.

B. Indications for Surgical Treatment

It should immediately be stipulated that these interventions, when carried out early enough and under good conditions—though they are not devoid of the risks inherent in any surgical procedure—are nevertheless minor operations. Statistics established on the basis of the literature show a 8.4% mortality rate. When reading the case reports, one becomes aware that the interventions are often carried out in severely disabled patients. By practising some prophylactic measures, the percentage

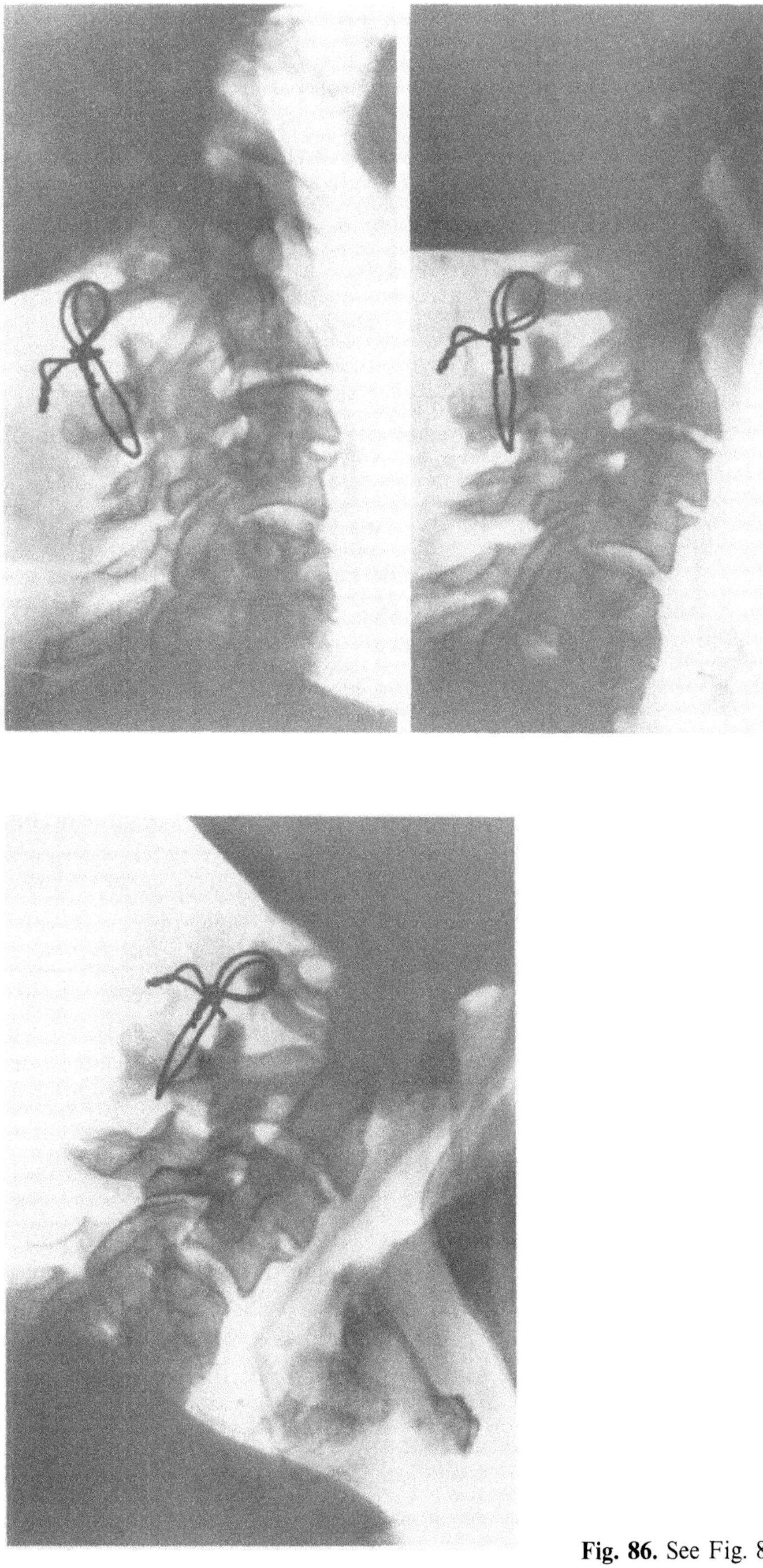

Fig. 86. See Fig. 84

could be lowered. Therefore, we recommend early surgery. What prevents the physicians from adopting a resolutely surgical attitude is the long immobilization period secondary to fusion. On the other hand, the absence of bone consolidation observed by us in three out of our five operated patients also accounts for some hesitation on our part. It seems possible that these two drawbacks can be eliminated by the utilization of acrylic cement or of osteosynthesis material allowing the patient to walk around without a plaster collar soon after operation. These new techniques make surgery the treatment of choice in lesions of the cervico-occipital joint.

C1/2 fusion is performed in about 18% of cases (Fig. 82). Indeed, though this technique has the advantage of only moderate limitation of mobility, the risk of pseudarthrosis and of absence of fusion of the bone graft is fairly high. On the other hand, C1/2 fusion does not, theoretically, secure the patient from any further neurologic complications. But atlantoaxial subluxations, which are only painful or accompanied by sensations of instability, failed to improve after treatment by external consolidation, may be retained as indications for this technique. However, we prefer the occipitoaxial fusion (Fig. 83).

It seems to us that this intervention should be performed in quite a number of conditions. Thus, atlantoaxial subluxation, which throughout three successive examinations is undisputably proved to be progressive and especially when it occurs in young subjects with well-preserved functional capacity, is in our opinion, an indication for arthrodesis of the cervico-occipital joint. This had been the case in one of our patients. The fast progressive erosion of the odontoid or of the anterior arch of the atlas (Figs. 13, 81) makes the patient run definite risks.

Though favorable courses have been described, it is safer to take steps to prevent a fatal outcome. Finally, the presence of neurological signs ascertained by several examiners, and, if need be, confirmed by positive contrast investigations, must always make surgery a consideration. In these cases, too, marked regression of the neurological signs following medical treatment has been reported, but the neurological symptomatology improves entirely only very rarely. Whether it is a matter of compression of the medulla oblongata or of vertebral artery insufficiency, surgery is justified.

Should the problem of indication of decompression remain, it is most often achieved by removal of the posterior arch of the atlas. Some, like Ickovic [181], recommend its systematic removal even in the absence of compression. They estimate that satisfactory reduction, or at least stable and definitive reduction of the subluxation, is never assured. Moreover, Ickovic thinks that removal of the posterior arch solves the problem of the indication for myelography. Myelography, according to him, is so harmful that it should be reserved only for cases with a discrepancy between the symptomatology and the data of the current radiological investigations, or when neurological symptoms persist or appear after the intervention. To support this position, he reports the case of a patient operated on for a subluxation of 12 mm without neurological signs but in whom, on account of the very destructive character of the rheumatoid arthritis, there was fear of a rapid development of the cervico-occipital lesion. The intervention showed the posterior arch of the atlas to clearly compress the upper segment of the spinal cord, especially on the right side. If myelography had been performed it would probably have shown this compression, but in its absence systematic removal of the anterior arch of the atlas permitted the eventual occurrence of neurological complications to be palliated. We believe that removal of the posterior arch of the atlas should not be systematic, but to be indicated when the intervention gives evidence of some compression, or when the diastasis is not entirely reduced.

There should be no more technically insolvable problems as concerns surgery of the cervico-occipital joint in chronic inflammatory rheumatism, save for some very specific major neurologic lesions. The operative indication, however, will remain moot, especially for physicians and rheumatologists who are not familiar with surgical techniques.

References

1. Ahlgren, P., Fog, J.: Atlanto-epistrophical subluxation in rheumatoid arthritis. Acta rheum. scand. **14**, 210–221 (1968)
2. Aita, J.A.: Neurologic manifestations of rheumatoid arthritis. Neb. med. J. **57**, 439–443 (1972)
3. Albers, D.: Eine Studie über die Funktion der HWS bei dorsaler und ventraler Flexion. Fortschr. Röntgenstr. **81**, 606 (1954)
4. Albertal, H.: Arthrosis occipitoatloidea y atloideaaxoidea. Sem. méd. (B. Aires) **122**, 670 (1963)
5. Albrecht, P.: La luxation spontanée de l'atlas sur l'axis chez l'adulte. Contribution à son étude clinique et radiologique. Thèse Genève, 1955, No. 47, p. 39
6. Alexander, E., Forsyth, H.F., Davis, C.H., Nashold, B.S.: Dislocation of atlas on axis: value of fusion of C 1, C 2 and C 3. J. Neurosurg. **15**, 353–371 (1958)
7. Ansell, B.N., Bywaters, E.G.L.: Growth in Still's disease. Ann. rheum. Dis. **15**, 295–319 (1956)
8. Ansell, B.N., Bywaters, E.G.L.: Radiological abnormalities in the cervical spine in juvenile rheumatoid arthritis. Xe Congrès de la Ligue internat. contre le Rhumatisme, Rome, 1961
9. Arlet, J., Andre, J., Dunglas, J., Vidal, R.: Luxation atloïdo-axoïdienne au cours de la polyarthrite chronique évolutive de l'adulte. A propos de 5 observations dont deux avec signes neurologiques. Rev. Rhum. **30**, 552–557 (1963)
10. Arlet, J., Pujol, M., Buc, A., Geraud, G., Gayrard, M., Latorzeff, S.: Rôle de l'hyperostose vertébrale dans les myélopathies cervicales. Rev. Rhum. **43**, 167–175 (1976)
11. Ashkenazy, H.M., Braham, J., Kozary, I.Z.: Delayed spinal myelopathy after atlanto-axial fracture dislocation. J. Neurosurg. **17**, 1100–1103 (1960)
12. Auquier, L., Paolaggi, J.B., Boddaert, P., Rouquès, C.: Spondylodiscite cervicale et compression médullaire opérée au cours d'une polyarthrite chronique séro-négative. Rôle favorisant possible d'une étroitesse du canal rachidien. Rev. Rhum. **35**, 542–544 (1974)
13. Auquier, L., Siaud, J.R., Guiot, G., Lhermitte, F.: Syndrome de la queue de cheval au cours de la spondylarthrite ankylosante. Découverte opératoire d'une fusion entre vertèbre et dure-mère dans le cas rapporté. Rev. Rhum. **41**, 733–737 (1974)
14. Babin, E.: La mesure du diamètre sagittal du canal cervical chez l'adulte. Sem. Hôp. Paris **46**, 2739–2742 (1970)
15. Baggenstoss, A.H., Bickel, W.H., Ward, L.E.: Rheumatoid granulomatous nodules as destructive lesions of vertebrae. J. Bone Jt Surg. **34A**, 601–609 (1952)
16. Bakay, L., Cares, H.L., Smith, R.J.: Ossification in the region of the posterior longitudinal ligament as cause of cervical myelopathy. J. Neurol. Neurosurg. Psychiat. **33**, 263–268 (1970)
17. Bakke, S.N.: Spondylosis ossificans ligamentosa localisata. Fortschr. Röntgenstr. **53**, 411–417 (1936)
18. Baleriaux, W.D., Jeanmart, L., Brihaye, J., Laurent-Montet, H.: Subluxation atloïdienne dans le cadre de la polyarthrite rhumatoïde. J. belge Rhum. Méd. phys. **30**, 222–227 (1975)
19. Ball, J.: Pathology of the rheumatoid cervical spine. Ann. rheum. Dis. **17**, 121 (1958)
20. Ball, J.: Mobility and instability in the cervical spine. J. Bone Jt Surg. **43B**, 600 (1961)
21. Barraquer-Tolosa, L., Barraquer-Ferre,

L., Duran, F., Madolell, A., Tolosa, E., Torruella-Pausa, J., Segara-Obiol, J.M.: Myélopathie très tardive consécutive à une fracture odontoïdienne avec luxation atlanto-axoïdienne. Rev. neurol. **89**, 193–207 (1953)

22. Barret, P.: Contribution à l'étude des luxations atloïdo-axoïdiennes au cours des polyarthrites rhumatoïdes de l'adulte. A propos de 4 observations personnelles. Thèse Grenoble, 1965, No. 9, p. 66
23. Bastin, J.M.: Intérêt de la photoscintigraphie au technetium dans le diagnostic de l'arthrite rhumatoïde du rachis cervical supérieur. J. belge Rhum. Méd. phys. **27**, 5–12 (1972)
24. Baumgartner, J.C.: Les localisations atloïdo-axoïdiennes de la spondylarthrite ankylosante. Mémoire C.E.S. Nancy, 1973, p. 22
25. Bell, C.: The nervous system of the human body. London: Longmans 1830
26. Beran, J., Suchomel, J.: Atlantoaxiálrú dislokace u progresívní polyartriady a Bechtěrovovy choroby. Čsl. Radiol. **22**, 9–17 (1968)
27. Berkheiser, E.J., Seidler, P.: Non traumatic dislocation of the atloido-axial joint. J. Amer. med. Ass. **96**, 517–523 (1931)
28. Berney, J., Taillard, W.: Transoral approach to the upper cervical spine and occipito-cervical spondylodesis in the cervical spine. 1st ed., pp. 217–225. Bern: Hans Huber 1974
29. Bertrand, J.: Contribution à l'étude clinique et radiologique de l'atteinte cervicale au cours de la polyarthrite rhumatoïde de l'adulte. Thèse Lyon, 1975, p. 81
30. Bied, J.C.: L'ostéoporose de la polyarthrite rhumatoïde. Thèse Lyon, 1966, No. 161, p. 66
31. Bland, J.H.: Rheumatoid arthritis of the cervical spine. Bull. rheum. Dis. **18**, 471–475 (1967)
32. Bland, J.H., Davis, P.H., Conlon, M.G., Van Buskirk, F.W., Duart, C.G.: Rheumatoid arthritis of cervical spine. Arch. intern. Med. **112**, 892–898 (1963)
33. Bland, J.H., Van Buskirk, F.W., Davis, P.H., Duart, C.G.: Rheumatoid arthritis of the cervical spine. Arthr. Rheum. **6**, 637–638 (1962)
34. Bland, J.H., Van Buskirk, F.W., Tamsa, J.P., Brown, E.W., Clayton, E.V.: A study of roentgenologic criteria of rheumatoid arthritis of the cervical spine. Amer. J. Roentgenol. **95**, 949–954 (1965)
35. Blecourt, J.J., Venestra, S.M.: Transverse lesion in a patient with juvenile rheumatoid arthritis caused by subluxation of some cervical vertebrae. Acta rheum. scand. **4**, 251–255 (1960)
36. Boever, F., Hennebert, P.: Les dislocations non traumatiques de la colonne vertébrale. Rev. Orthop. **39**, 24–69 (1953)
37. Böger, A.: Ein Fall von Malum suboccipitale rheumaticum. Arch. orthop. u. Unfall-Chir. **3**, 97–100 (1905)
38. Boldrey, C.E., Maass, L., Miller, F.: The role of atlantoid compression in the etiology of internal carotid thrombosis. J. Neurosurg. **13**, 127 (1956)
39. Bonnet, J.R.: Contribution à l'étude clinique et radiologique de la colonne cervicale dans la polyarthrite chronique rhumatismale. Mémoire C.E.S. Rhumatologie, Paris, 1961, p. 50
40. Bonney, G.: Stabilization of the upper cervical spine by transpharyngeal route. Proc. roy. Soc. Med. **63**, 896–897 (1970)
41. Bontoux, D., Alcalay, K., Nolen, P.: Luxations cervicales multiples et tétraplégie au cours d'une polyarthrite rhumatoïde. Sci. Med. **5**, 319–329 (1974)
42. Boogaard, J.A.: De indrukking der grandvlakte van de Schedel door de vervelkolom, har oorzaken en gevolzen. Ned. T. Geneesk. **2**, 81 (1865)
43. Bourgeois, H., Grisel, P.: Un nouveau cas de torticolis naso-pharyngien. Presse méd. **1931**, 722
44. Bowie, E.A., Glasgow, G.I.: Cauda equina lesions associated with ankylosing spondylitis: report of three cases. Brit. med. J. **1961 II**, 24–27
45. Boyle, A.C.: The rheumatoid neck. Proc. roy. Soc. Med. **64**, 1161–1968 (1971)
46. Brattström, M.: Traitement des luxations atloïdo-axoïdiennes au cours de la polyarthrite rhumatoïde. Abstracts of the VII European Rheumatology Congress, 1971, Brighton, Symposium 31
47. Brattström, M., Elner, Å., Granholm, L.: Transoral surgery for myelopathy caused by rheumatoid arthritis of the cervical spine. Ann. rheum. Dis. **32**, 578–581 (1973)

48. Brattström, M., Granholm, L.: Chirurgie der Halswirbelsäule bei Patienten mit rheumatoider Arthritis. Orthopäde **2**, 118–120 (1973)
49. Brattström, M., Granholm, L.: Operative treatment of atlanto-axial luxation in rheumatoid arthritis. VIII European Rheumatology Congress, Helsinki 1975. Scand. J. Rheum., Suppl. **8**, 009
50. Briedal, P.: Ossification of the posterior longitudinal ligament in the cervical spine. "The Japanese Disease" occurring in patients of British Descent. Aust. Radiol. **13**, 311–313 (1969)
51. Brinkmann, E.: Die Drehungsverrenkung des Atlas. Klin. Wschr. **7**, 649–650 (1928)
52. Brocher, J.E.W.: Die Occipito-cervicalgegend. Stuttgart: Thieme 1954
53. Bruhin, A., Wagenhauser, F.J.: Der Befall der Halswirbelsäule bei der progredient chronischen Polyarthritis. Schweiz. med. Wschr. **101**, 277–279 (1971)
54. Buetti-Bäuml, C.: Funktionelle Röntgendiagnostik der Halswirbelsäule. Stuttgart: Thieme 1954
55. Bywaters, E.G.L., Ansell, B.M., Wood, Ph.N.: Nomenclature and classification of juvenile chronic polyarthritis. Scand. J. Rheum., Suppl. **8**, 34-02, 34-03 (1975)
56. Bywaters, E.G.L., Dixon, A.S.: Paravertebral ossifications in psoriatic arthritis. Ann. rheum. Dis. **24**, 313 (1965)
57. Capra, R., Secondo, G.: Su un caso di spondilodiscite in poliartrite cronica. Reumatismo **21**, 110–113 (1969)
58. Car, A.: Promjene na cervikalnoj kičmi u tokn ankilozantnoy spondilitisa kod našif bolesnica. Reumatizam **17**, 169–175 (1970)
59. Carlioz, H., Dubousset, J.: Les instabilités entre l'atlas et l'axis chez l'enfant. Rev. Chir. orthop. **59**, 291 (1973)
60. Caslo, G., Fontana, G.: La colonna vertebrale nell'artrite reumatoida. Reumatisma **17**, 325–335 (1965)
61. Castaigne, P., Cambier, J., Escourolle, R., Masson, M., Berger, B.: Etude anatomoclinique d'un cas de spondylarthrite ankylosante compliquée d'un syndrome de la moelle dorsale. Bull. Soc. méd. Hôp. Paris **116**, 321–327 (1965)
62. Castaigne, P., Escourolle, R., Brunet, P., Hauw, J.J., Ricou, P., Truelle, J.L.: Déterminations inflammatoires nerveuses et musculaires squelettiques et myocardiques, au cours d'une maladie rhumatoïde. Ann. Méd. Interne (Paris) **125**, 177–183 (1975)
63. Castaing, J., Gonaze, E., Plisson, J.: Technique de l'arthrodèse cervico-occipitale par greffon vissé dans l'occipital. Rev. Chir. orthop. **49**, 721–726 (1972)
64. Chand, K.: Cervical spine and rheumatoid arthritis. Int. Surg. **57**, 721–726 (1972)
65. Chaouat, Y.: Les atteintes cervicales dans la polyarthrite rhumatoïde de l'adulte. In: Progrès en rhumatologie, pp. 31–38. Paris: Flammarion 1968
66. Chaouat, Y.: Les polyarthrites de l'enfant. Les rhumatismes chroniques inflammatoires de l'enfant. In: Progrès en rhumatologie, pp. 67–83. Paris: Flammarion 1968
67. Chaouat, Y., Kanovitch, J.: Les malformations de la charnière. A propos de 7 observations découvertes dans un service de rhumatologie. Rev. Rhum. **39**, 115 (1972)
68. Charbonnel, Farges, Lafite-Dupont: Arthrites cervicales et torticolis naso-pharyngien. Presse méd. 668 (1931)
69. Cibert, M.: Les luxations atloïdo-axoïdiennes au cours de la polyarthrite rhumatoïde de l'adulte. A propos de 27 cas, dont 7 opérés de greffe cervicale postérieure. Thèse Lyon, 1969, No. 160, p. 136
70. Cibert, M., Vignon, G., Chapuy, P.: La luxation atloïdo-axoïdienne au cours de la polyarthrite de l'adulte. A propos de 27 cas, dont 7 opérés de greffe cervicale postérieure. Rev. lyon. Méd. **19**, 77–92 (1970)
71. Claessens, M.I., Redant, W.A., Veys, E.N.: De atlanto-epistrofeal luxatie bij reumatoide artritis. T. Geneesk. **16**, 1065–1069 (1972)
72. Cohen, C.: Luxation fatale du rachis cervical dans la polyarthrite rhumatoïde. Geront. Clin. **11**, 239–243 (1969)
73. Conlon, P.W.: The cervical spine in rheumatoid arthritis. Clin. Med. **74**, 29–36 (1967)
74. Conlon, P.W., Isdale, I.C., Rose, B.S.: Some unusual lesions of the cervical spine in rheumatoid arthritis. N.Z. med. J. **62**, 279–283 (1963)
75. Conlon, P.W.,. Isdale, I.C., Rose, B.S.: Rheumatoid arthritis of the cervical spine.

An analysis of 333 cases. Ann. rheum. Dis. **25**, 120–126 (1966)
76. Corrigan, A.B.: Radiological changes in rheumatoid cervical spines. Aust. Radiol. **13**, 370–375 (1969)
77. Coss, J.A., Jr., Boots, R.M.: Juvenile rheumatoid arthritis. A study of fifty-six cases with a note on skeletal changes. J. Pediat. **29**, 143–156 (1946)
78. Coste, F., Auquier, L., Civatte, J.: Polyarthrite chronique évolutive avec luxation atloïdo-axoïdienne, sans signe de compression médullaire. Rev. Rhum. **19**, 55–56 (1952)
79. Coste, F., Delbarre, F., Cayla, J., Lambert, P.: Remarques sur la luxation des vertèbres cervicales dans la polyarthrite rhumatoïde. Sem. Hôp. Paris **36**, 1121–1130 (1960)
80. Coste, F., Merle d'Aubigne, R., Garcin, R.: Troubles bulbaires paroxystiques par luxation antérieure atloïdo-occipitale dans une spondylarthrite ankylosante. Résultat favorable d'une greffe postérieure. Sem. Hôp. Paris. **36**, 1130–1133 (1960)
81. Coutts, M.B.: Atlanto-epistropheal subluxations. Arch. Surg. (Chic.) **29**, 297–311 (1934)
82. Cregan, J.C.F.: Internal fixation of the unstable rheumatoid cervical spine. Ann. rheum. Dis. **25**, 242–252 (1966)
83. Crellin, R.Q., Maccabe, J.J., Hamilton, E.B.D.: Severe subluxation of the cervical spine in rheumatoid arthritis. J. Bone Jt Surg. **52B**, 244–251 (1970)
84. Crespo-Vaquez, A.: Le rachis cervical dans la polyarthrite rhumatoïde de l'adulte. Mémoire d'assistant étranger, Paris, 1967, No. 24, p. 113
85. Creyssel, J., Ravault, P.P., Vignon, C., Mourgues, G. de, Fischer, L.: Incidence chirurgicale dans les luxations atloïdo-axoïdiennes et les ostéolyses de l'apophyse odontoïde au cours de la polyarthrite rhumatoïde et de la spondylarthrite ankylosante. Rhumatologie **21**, 293–302 (1969)
86. Cuevillas, A.R.L.: Otzo caso de luxacion patologica del axis. Bol. Soc. argent. Ortop. Traum. **26**, 2–7 (1961)
87. Dally: Du torticolis occipito-atloïdien. Bull. gen. Thér., Paris, 1975, 354–356
88. David-Chaussé, J., Dehais, J., Bourde, J.C.: Manifestations vertébrales douloureuses et chondrocalcinose articulaire diffuse. Rev. Rhum. **40**, 635–642 (1973)
89. Davis, F.W., Markley, M.E.: Rheumatoid arthritis with death from medullary compression. Ann. intern. Med. **35**, 451–454 (1951)
91. Debeyre, J., Sterboul, A.: Une technique d'arthrodèse occipito-atloïdienne. Rev. Rhum. **18**, 10–12 (1951)
92. Debeyre, N.: Le rachis cervical dans la polyarthrite rhumatoïde de l'adulte. Feuill. Prat. **35**, 209–214 (1970)
93. Decoulx, P.: Mobilité du rachis cervical. Evolution clinique. Nouv. Presse méd. **2**, 657–659 (1973)
94. Delgoffe, A.: La soi-disant énucléation de l'atlas et le torticolis. Rev. Orthop. **21**, 5–12 (1934)
95. Desfosses, P.: Un cas de maladie de Grisel. Torticolis naso-pharyngien par subluxation de l'atlas. Presse méd. 1179–1180 (1930)
96. Detenbeck, L.C.: Rheumatoid arthritis of the spinal column. Pathological aspects and treatment. Orthop. Clin. N. Amer. **2**, 679–686 (1971)
97. Di Chiro, G., Fischer, R.L.: Contrast radiography of the spinal cord. Arch. Neurol. (Paris) **11**, 125 (1964)
98. Dihlmann, W.: Spondylitis ankylopoetica. Die Bechterewsche Krankheit. Stuttgart: Thieme 1968
99. Dirheimer, Y.: Impression basilaire et polyarthrite rhumatoïde. Sem. Hôp. Paris **50**, 2067–2072 (1974)
100. Dirheimer, Y.: L'utilisation du phosphore en rhumatologie. J. méd. Strasbourg **6**, 99–108 (1975)
101. Dirheimer, Y., Babin, E.: Basilar impression and hereditary fragility of the bone. Neuroradiology **3**, 41–43 (1971)
102. Dirheimer, Y., Babin, E.: Upward atlanto-axial dislocation in rheumatoid arthritis. Neuroradiology **7**, 229–236 (1974)
103. Dirheimer, Y., Grosshans, E., Haller, H., Ramsheyi, A., Ramsheyi, M., Reolon, M.: Les lésions d'hyperostose de la charnière cervico-occipitale au cours du psoriasis et des arthropathies psoriasiques (to be published)
104. Dirheimer, Y., Ramsheyi, A., Reolon, M.: Positive arthrography of the cranio-cervical joints. Neuroradiology **12**, 257–260 (1977)

105. Dirheimer, Y., Wackenheim, A.: Etude radiologique des localisations de l'hyperostose vertébrale au niveau de la charnière cervico-occipitale. Sem. Hôp. Paris **46**, 2734–2738 (1970)
106. Dirheimer, Y., Wackenheim, A.: L'apophyse odontoïde couronnée. A propos du mécanisme de développement de certaines images de manifestations de la vertèbre occipitale. Sem. Hôp. Paris **50**, 2077–2080 (1974)
107. Djian, A., Debeyre, N., Sèze, S. de: Les atteintes de la charnière cervico-occipitale au cours de la polyarthrite rhumatoïde. In: L'Actualité rhumatologique. Paris: Expansion scientifique française (édit.) 1966
108. Djian, A., Zinn, W.: Der Wert der funktionellen Röntgenuntersuchung des Gelenkes zwischen erstem und zweiten Halswirbel. Z. Rheumaforsch. **18**, 279–291 (1959)
109. Dryll, A., Cazalis, P., Debeyre, N., Sèze, S. de: Rhumatisme psoriasique. Etude prospective de 50 cas, sans atteinte sacroiliaque et sans facteur rhumatoïde, appariés à 50 cas de polyarthrites rhumatoïdes. Nouv. Presse méd. **4**, 1408–1412 (1975)
110. Dryll, A., Kuntz, D., Sèze, S. de: Etude comparative de 35 cas de pelvispondylite psoriasique appariés à 35 cas de pelvispondylite rhumatismale. Sem. Hôp. Paris **49**, 2439–2444 (1973)
111. Dubousset, J., Ramon-Soler, R., Ramadier, J.O.: Arthrodèses de la région crânio-rachidienne. Rev. Chir. orthop. **55**, 29–54 (1969)
112. Dunbar, H.S., Rays, B.S.: Chronic atlanto-axial dislocations with late neurologic manifestations. Surg. Gynec. Obstet. **113**, 757–762 (1961)
113. Duyfjes, F.: Occipito-cervical spondylodesis for atlanto-axial instability with neurological changes in rheumatoid conditions. Acta orthop. belg. **38**, 40–46 (1972)
114. Edström, G.: Rheumatoid arthritis and Still's disease in children. A survey of 161 cases. Arthr. Rheum. **1**, 499–504 (1958)
115. Ely, L.W.: Subluxation of the atlas. Report of two cases. Ann. Surg. **54**, 20–29 (1911)
116. Englander, D.: Non traumatic occipito-atlanto-axial dislocation. Contribution to the radiology of atlas. Brit. J. Radiol. **15**, 341–346 (1942)
117. Ettmann, I.N.: Agenesis of the odontoid with chronic subluxation of the atlanto-axial joint. J. Tenn. Med. Ass. **57**, 438–441 (1964)
118. Eulderink, F., Meijers, K.A.E.: Pathological changes in the C 1–C 2 area in the cervical spine in rheumatoid arthritis. Abstracts of the VII European Rheumatology Congress, 1971, Brighton 38-2
119. Eulderink, F., Meijers, K.A.E.: Pathology of the cervical spine in rheumatoid arthritis. VIII European Rheumatology Congress, Helsinki, 1975. Scand. J. Rheum. Suppl. **8**, 063
120. Evans, W.: Pathologic dislocations at the atlanto-axial joint: an unusual complication of rheumatic fever. Radiology **37**, 347–350 (1941)
121. Fang, M.S.Y., Ong, G.B.: Direct anterior approach to the upper cervical spine. J. Bone Jt Surg. **44A**, 1588–1604 (1962)
122. Farhat, S.M., Schneider, R.C., Gray, J.M.: Traumatic spinal extradural hematoma associated with cervical fractures in rheumatoid spondylitis. J. Traum. **13**, 591–599 (1973)
123. Felten, M.: Über Atlasluxationen. Z. Orthop. **89**, 293–309 (1958)
124. Ferguson, R.H., Slocumb, C.M.: Peripheral neuropathy in rheumatoid arthritis. Bull. rheum. Dis. **11**, 252 (1961)
125. Fick, H.: Handbuch der Anatomie und Mechanik der Gelenke. (Tome 3.) Jena: Fischer 1911
126. Finger, H., Kikillus, B.: Atlanto-epistropheale Luxation als komplizierendes Symptom chronisch rheumatischer Erkrankungen. Dtsch. med. Wschr. **89**, 1546–1549 (1964)
127. Fitzwilliams, D.C.L.: Inflammatory dislocation of the atlas. Brit. med. J. **1934II**, 107–109
128. Force, L., Castera, J., Herne, N., Navarranne, P.: Luxation atloïdo-axoïdienne mortelle au cours d'une polyarthrite rhumatoïde. Marseille méd. **104**, 697–699 (1967)
129. Forestier, J., Certonciny, A., Faidherbe, P., Djian, A.: Atteinte de la charnière cervico-occipitale au cours d'une forme ostéolytique de polyarthrite chronique évolutive

avec quadriplégie. Rev. Rhum. **30**, 557–559 (1963)

130. Forestier, J., Jacqueline, F., Rotes-Querol, J.: La spondylarthrite ankylosante. Paris: Masson 1961
131. Forestier, J., Lagier, R.: Ankylosing hyperostosis of the spine. Clin. Orthop. **74**, 65–83 (1971)
132. Forestier, J., Rozier, M.: Subluxation cervicale au cours d'une spondylarthrite ankylosante. Rhumatologie **4**, 186–188 (1949)
133. Forsyth, H.F., Alexandre, E., Davis, C., Underdal, R.: The advantage of early spine fusion in the fracture-dislocation of the cervical spine. J. Bone Jt Surg. **41A**, 17–36 (1959)
134. Fränkel, E.: Über chronisch ankylosierende Wirbelsäulenversteifung. Fortschr. Röntgenstr. **7**, 62 (1903/1904)
135. Fränkel, E.: Über chronisch ankylosierende Wirbelsäulenversteifung. Fortschr. Röntgenstr. **11**, 171 (1907)
136. Freehafer, A.A., Weiss, L.S.: Atraumatic subluxation and dislocation of the cervical spine in rheumatoid arthritis. Arthr. Rheum. **7**, 308 (1964)
137. Friedman, H.: Intraspinal rheumatoid nodule causing nerve root compression: case report. J. Neurosurg. **32**, 689–691 (1970)
138. Garcin, R., Godlewski, S., Postel, M., Dry, J.: Sur une invagination axoïdo-atloïdienne (ascension de l'axis à travers l'atlas) avec algies occipitales rebelles au cours d'une polyarthrite chronique évolutive, évoluant depuis 25 ans. Résultats de la greffe osseuse postérieure. Rev. neurol. **102**, 486–494 (1960)
139. Garcin, R., Godlewski, S., Robain, O., Dry, J.: Sur une ataxie par troubles de la sensibilité profonde au cours d'une polyarthrite rhumatoïde évoluant depuis 10 ans. Découverte radiologique d'une luxation atloïdo-axoïdienne. Rev. Rhum. **30**, 570–571 (1963)
140. Garrod, A.E.: A treatise on rheumatism and rheumatoid arthritis. London: C. Griffin and Co. 1890
141. Giuliano, V.J., Scully, T.J.: Atlanto-axial subluxation in psoriatic arthropathy. Arch. Derm. (Chic.) **105**, 247–248 (1972)
142. Gleason, I.O., Urist, M.R.: Atlanto-axial dislocation with odontoid separation in rheumatoid disease. Clin. Orthop. **42**, 121–129 (1965)
143. Godlewski, S.: Quelques apports récents sur les anomalies congénitales de la charnière cervico-occipitale. Sem. Hôp. Paris **48**, 1635–1679 (1972)
144. Gordon, A.L., Yudell, A.: Cauda equina lesion associated with rheumatoid spondylitis. Ann. intern. Med. **78**, 555–557 (1973)
145. Gounelle, M., Marche, J.: La maladie rhumatismale post-dysentérique. Rev. Rhum. **8**, 355 (1941)
146. Goutelle, A., Dejour, H., Megard, M., Bouvier, M., Cibert, M., Brunon, J., Marsan, C.: Le traitement chirurgical des luxations atloïdo-axoïdiennes d'origine rhumatismale. J. Med. Lyon **51**, 1895–1904 (1970)
147. Graham, D.C.: Spontaneous atlanto-axial subluxation in rheumatoid arthritis and ankylosing spondylitis. Arthr. Rheum. **3**, 446–447 (1960)
148. Gray, H., Goss, C.M.: Anatomy of the human body. 28th ed. Philadelphia: Lea and Febiger 1966
149. Greenberg, A.D.: Atloido-axoidal dislocation. Brain **91**, 655–684 (1968)
150. Greig, D.M.: Clinical observations on the surgical pathology of bone. Edinburgh and London: Oliver and Boyd 1931
151. Grisel, P.: Enucléation de l'atlas et torticolis naso-pharyngien. Presse méd. 50-53 (1930)
152. Grisel, P., Bourgeois, H.: Un nouveau cas de torticolis naso-pharyngien. Ann. Otolaryng. (Paris) 725–731 (1931)
153. Grisolia, A., Bell, R.L., Peltier, L.F.: Fractures and dislocations of the spine complicating spondylitis. A report of six cases. J. Bone Jt Surg. **49A**, 339–344 (1967)
154. Grogono, B.J.S.: Injuries of the atlas and axis. J. Bone Jt Surg. **36B**, 397–410 (1954)
155. Grokoest, A.W., Snyder, A.I., Schlaeger, R.: Juvenile rheumatoid arthritis, p. 120. Boston: Little, Brown 1962
156. Gros, C., Rollgen, A., Vlahovitch, B.: Manifestations neurologiques des luxations non traumatiques atloïdo-axoïdiennes. Neurochirurgie **6**, 197–204 (1960)
157. Gros, C.M., Wackenheim, A.: Critère radiologique de l'impression basilaire. J. Radiol. Électrol. **45**, 781–788 (1964)
158. Guillaume, J.: L'ostéosynthèse métallique

dans les luxations de l'atlas. Rev. neurol. **85**, 513–515 (1952)
159. Gutmann, L., Hable, K.: Rheumatoid pachymeningitis. Neurology (Minneap.) **13**, 901–905 (1963)
160. Hadley, L.A.: Roentgenographic studies of the cervical spine. Amer. J. Roentgenol. **52**, 173 (1944)
161. Hadley, L.A.: Atlanto-occipital fusion, osiculum terminale, occipital vertebra as related to basilar impression with neurological symptoms. Amer. J. Roentgenol. **59**, 511 (1948)
162. Hamblen, D.L.: Occipito-cervical fusion. Indications, technic and results. J. Bone Jt Surg. **49B**, 33–45 (1967)
163. Hart, F.D.: Extra-articular manifestations of rheumatoid arthritis. Semin. Arthr. Rheum. **1**, 161–173 (1971)
164. Hart, F.D.: Rheumatoid arthritis: extra-articular manifestations. I. Brit. med. J. **1969III**, 131
165. Hart, F.D.: Rheumatoid arthritis: extra-articular manifestations. II. Brit. med. J. **1970II**, 747
166. Hart, F.D., Golding, J.R.: Rheumatoid neuropathy. Brit. med. J. **1960I**, 1594
167. Hauge, T.: So-called spontanous cervical dislocation. A clinical, roentgenological, surgical and post-mortem study on the pathogeny and treatment in five cases. Acta clin. scand., Suppl. **232**, 1–28 (1958)
168. Hauge, T.: Chronic rheumatoid polyarthritis and spondylarthritis associated with neurological symptoms and signs occasionally simulating an intraspinal expansive process. Acta chir. scand. **120**, 395–401 (1961)
169. Hecker, P.: Appareil ligamenteux-occipito-atloïdo-axoïdien. Etude d'anatomie comparée. Arch. Anat. (Strasbourg) **1**, 413–436 (1922); **2**, 57–96 (1923)
170. Henderson, D.R.F.: Vertical atlanto-axial subluxation in rheumatoid arthritis. Rheum. Rehab. **14**, 31–38 (1975)
171. Henocq, A., Deshayes, P., Menibus, C.H., Dailly, R.: La radiologie dans la polyarthrite juvénile. A propos de 26 observations de maladie de Still. Ouest méd. **25**, 399–408 (1972)
172. Henrard, J.C.: Contribution à l'étude de la polyarthrite rhumatoïde. A propos de 100 polyarthrites rhumatoïdes féminines ayant débuté à l'âge adulte. Thèse Paris, 1968, No. 749, p. 152.
173. Hess, J.H., Bronstein, I.P., Abelson, S.M.: Atlanto-axial dislocations associated, with trauma and secondary to inflammatory foci in the neck. Amer. J. Dis. Child. **49**, 1137–1147 (1935)
174. Hinck, V.C., Hopkins, C.E.: Measurement of atlantodental interval in adult. Amer. J. Roentgenol. **84**, 945–951 (1960)
175. Hohl, M., Baker, M.R.: The atlanto-axial joint. Roentgenographic and anatomical study of normal and abnormal motion. J. Bone Jt Surg. **46A**, 1739–1752 (1964)
176. Hohmann, D.: Spontane atlanto-axiale Ventralluxation bei Spondylarthritis ankylopoetica mit intermittierenden Lähmungen. Arch. orthop. Unfall-Chir. **59**, 56–65 (1966)
177. Hohmann, D., Walcher, K.: Röntgenologisch funktionelle Studien der Atlanto-Okzipital-Region bei Spondylarthritis ankylopoetica. Z. Orthop. **103**, 5–23 (1967)
178. Hollin, S.H., Gross, W.W.. Levin, P.: Fracture of the cervical spine in patients with rheumatoid disease. Amer. Surg. **71**, 532–536 (1956)
179. Holzmann, H., Hoede, N., Eissner, D., Mahn, K., Hulse, R.: Joint involvement in psoriasis. Arch. derm. Forsch. **250**, 95–107 (1974)
180. Hopkins, J.S.: Lower cervical rheumatoid subluxation with tetraplegia. J. Bone Jt Surg. **49B**, 46–51 (1967)
181. Ickovic, B.: Les luxations atloïdo-axoïdiennes dans la polyarthrite rhumatoïde et la spondylarthrite ankylosante. Les complications neurologiques. Les résultats et les indications de la chirurgie de fixation. Mémoire CES Rhumato, Paris 1972, pp. 142
182. Isdale, I.C., Conlon, P.W.: Atlanto-axial subluxation. A six year follow up report. Ann. rheum. Dis. **40**, 387–389 (1971)
183. Isdale, I.C., Corrigan, A.B.: Backward luxation of the atlas. Two cases of an uncommon condition. Ann. rheum. Dis. **29**, 6–9 (1970)
184. Jackson, H.: The diagnosis of minimal atlanto-axial subluxation. Brit. J. Radiol. **23**, 672–674 (1950)
185. Jacobs, C.N.: Atlas and axis luxation. Amer. J. orthop. Surg. **16**, 357–364 (1918)

186. Jellinger, Y.: Rückenmarkbeteiligung bei Panarteritis nodosa. Beitr. path. Anat. **129**, 1–31 (1963)
187. Jirout, J.: Studies in the dynamics of the spine. Acta radiol. (Stockh.) **46**, 55–60 (1956)
188. Jirout, J.: Studien der Dynamik der Halswirbelsäule in der frontalen und horizontalen Ebene. Fortschr. Röntgenstr. **106**, 236–240 (1967)
189. Jung, D.: Os odontoïdeum et pseudarthrose de l'apophyse odontoïde. Diagnostic différentiel par les radiographies fonctionnelles de flexion-extension cervicales. Thèse Strasbourg, 1975, No. 98, p. 43
190. Kao, C.C., Messert, B., Winkler, S., Turner, J.H.: Rheumatoid C1-C2 dislocation: pathogenesis and treatment reconsidered. J. Neurol. Neurosurg. Psychiat. **37**, 1069–1073 (1974)
191. Kapandji, I.A.: Physiologie articulaire. Tome III: tronc et rachis, p. 255. Paris: Librairie Maloine 1972
192. Kaplan, D., Plotz, C.M., Nathason, L., Frank, L.: Cervical spine in psoriasis and in psoriatic arthritis. Ann. rheum. Dis. **23**, 5056 (1964)
193. Kersley, D.: Un cas unique de goutte. Rev. Rhum. **17**, 632–634 (1950)
194. Khilnani, M.T., Wolf, B.S.: Transverse diameter of cervical spinal cord in pantopaque myelography. J. Neurosurg. **20**, 660 (1963)
195. Kicevac-Miljkovic, A.: Radiological changes in cervical occipital joints during course of juvenile rheumatoid arthritis. Acta med. jugosl. **28**, 311–319 (1974)
196. Knese, K.H.: Kopfgelenk, Kopfhaltung und Kopfbewegung des Menschen. Z. Anat. Entwickl.-Gesch. **114**, 67–107 (1947)
197. Kopera, Z., Barwick-Schramm, A.: Dislocation of atlas during course of rheumatoid arthritis. Pol. Tyg. lek. **15**, 315–319 (1960)
198. Kornblum, D., Clayton, L., Nash, H.H.: Non traumatic cervical dislocation in rheumatoid spondylitis. J. Amer. med. Ass. **149**, 431–435 (1952)
199. Kotscher, E.: Spontane Subluxation im Atlanto-Axialgelenk bei entzündlichen Prozessen am Halse. Radiol. Clin. **24**, 17 (1955)
200. Kushner, I., Segel, A.: Rheumatoid involvement of the cervical spine; neurological manifestations and cineradiographic findings. XIe Congrès Internat. Maladies Rhumatismales, Mar del Plata 1965, Buenos-Aires, Yuste Publicidad, p. 251
201. Lambert, P.: Les luxations spontanées du rachis cervical. Rhumatologie **12**, 102–117 (1960)
202. Lawrence, J.S., Sharp, J., Ball, J., Bier, F.: Rheumatoid arthritis of the lumbar spine. Ann. rheum. Dis. **23**, 205–217 (1964)
203. Le Baudour, J.: Les localisations cervicales de la P.C.E. de l'enfant. Rhumatologie **9**, 60–71 (1957)
204. Le Baudour, J., Freyberg, R.H.: Contribution à l'étude de la polyarthrite chronique évolutive de l'enfant: ses localisations cervicales. Sem. Hôp. Paris **34**, 1120–1129 (1958)
205. Lee, M.L.R., Waters, M.J.: Neurological complications of ankylosing spondylitis. Brit. med. J. **1962I**, 798
206. Lemmen, L.J., Laing, P.G.: Fracture of the cervical spine in patients with rheumatoid arthritis. J. Neurosurg. **16**, 542–550 (1959)
207. Lewitt, K.: Blockierung von Atlas, Axis und Atlas, Okziput, in Röntgenbild und Klinik. Z. Orthop. **108**, 43–50 (1970)
208. Lewitt, K., Krausova, L.: Messungen in Vor- und Rückbeugen in den Kopfgelenken. Fortschr. Röntgenstr. **99**, 538 (1963)
209. Lewitt, K., Krausova, L.: Mechanismus und Bewegungsausmaß in den Kopfgelenken bei passiven Bewegungen. Z. Orthop. **103**, 323–333 (1967)
210. Lindgren, L., Ljunggren, B., Ratcheson, R.A.: Reposition, anterior exposure and fusion in the treatment on myelopathy caused by rheumatoid arthritis of the cervical spine. Report of 3 cases. Scand. J. Rheum. **3**, 195–199 (1974)
211. Lipscombs, P.R.: Cervico-occipital fusion for congenital and post-traumatic anomalies of the atlas and the axis. J. Bone Jt Surg. **39A**, 1289–1301 (1957)
212. Locke, G.R., Gardner, J.I., Van Epps, E.F.: Atlas-Dens Interval (A.D.I.) in children. A survey based on 200 normal cervical spines. Amer. J. Roentgenol. **97**, 135–140 (1966)
213. Lockie, L.M., Norcross, B.M.: Juvenile rheumatoid arthritis. Pediatrics **2**, 694–698 (1948)

214. Lombardi, G.: The occipital vertebra. Amer. J. Roentgenol. **86**, 260–269 (1961)
215. Losada, A., Ronban, E., Diaz, N.: Estudio clinico y radiologico de la columna cervical in artritis reumatoidea. Rev. méd. Chile **98**, 600–609 (1970)
216. Lounavaara, K.I.: Foreward subluxation of the atlas following birth trauma. Acta paediat. **37**, 340–348 (1949)
217. Lourie, M., Stewart, W.A.: Spontaneous atlanto-axial dislocation: a complication of rheumatoid disease. New Engl. J. Med. **265**, 677–681 (1961)
218. Mabon, R.F., Lowell, W.W.: Spontaneous atlanto-axial subluxation accompanied by severe neurologic defects. Surgery **40**, 770–777 (1956)
219. Magora, A., Wolf, E., Gonen, B.: Electrodiagnostic investigation of the neuromuscular lesions in rheumatoid arthritis. Acta rheum. scand. **16**, 280–292 (1970)
220. Maher, J.A.: Dural nodules in rheumatoid arthritis. Report of a case. Arch. Path. (Chic.) **58**, 354–359 (1954)
221. Malgaigne, J.F.: Traité des fractures et des luxations, Vol. II. Paris 1855
222. Margulies, M.E., Katz, J., Rosenberg, M.: Spontaneous dislocation of atlanto-axial joint in rheumatoid spondylitis: recovery from quadriplegia following surgical decompression. Neurology (Minneap.) **5**, 290–294 (1955)
223. Martel, W.: The occipito-atlanto-axial joints in rheumatoid arthritis and ankylosing spondylitis. Amer. J. Roentgenol. **86**, 223–240 (1961)
224. Martel, W.: Occipito-atlanto-axial joints in rheumatoid arthritis. Radiological aspects of rheumatoid arthritis. Proceedings of an International Symposium. International Congress series No. 61, p. 189. Amsterdam: Excerpta Medica Foundation 1963
225. Martel, W.: Cervical spondylitis in rheumatoid disease. A comment on neurologic significance and pathogenesis. Amer. J. Med. **44**, 441–446 (1968)
226. Martel, W., Abell, M.R.: Fatal atlanto-axial luxation in rheumatoid arthritis. Arthr. Rheum. **6**, 224–231 (1963)
227. Martel, W., Bole, G.G.: Pathologic fracture of the odontoid process in rheumatoid arthritis. Radiology **90**, 948–952 (1968)
228. Martel, W., Duff, I.F., Preston, R.H., Hayes, J.T.: The cervical spine in rheumatoid arthritis; correlation of radiographic and clinical manifestations. Arthr. Rheum. **7**, 326 (1964)
229. Martel, W., Holt, J.F., Cassidy, J.T.A.: Roentgenologic manifestation of juvenile rheumatoid arthritis. Amer. J. Roentgenol. **88**, 400–423 (1962)
230. Martel, W., Page, J.W.: Cervical vertebral erosion and subluxation in rheumatoid arthritis and ankylosing spondylitis. Arthr. Rheum. **3**, 546–556 (1960)
231. Martinez, S.N., Poirier, N., Papineau, L.T.: Luxation spontanée de l'atlas sur l'axis d'origine rhumatoïde. Un. méd. Can. **101**, 1544–1551 (1972)
232. Mason, B.M., Murray, R.S., Oates, J.K., Young, A.C.: A comparative radiological study of Reiter's disease, rheumatoid arthritis and ankylosing spondylitis. J. Bone Jt Surg. **41 B**, 137 (1959)
233. Mathews, J.A.: Atlanto-axial subluxation in rheumatoid arthritis. Ann. rheum. Dis. **28**, 260–266 (1969)
234. Mathews, J.A.: The pathogenesis of placid arm weakness in rheumatoid cervical myelopathy. VIII European Rheumatology Congress, Helsinki 1975. Scand. J. Rheum., Suppl. **8**, 064
235. Matthews, W.B.: The neurological complications of ankylosing spondylitis. J. neurol. Sci. **6**, 561–573 (1968)
236. Matzdorf, M.: Röntgenuntersuchungen über die Bedeutung der Atlasregion als Krankheitsfaktor. Z. Orthop. **87**, 165 (1956)
237. Mazare, Y., Jacquot, F., Nicoud, M., Phelip, X., Barret, P.: Les luxations atloïdo-axoïdiennes au cours des polyarthrites rhumatoïdes de l'adulte. A propos de 5 observations. Rev. lyon. Méd. **16**, 209–218 (1967)
238. McEwen, C., Ditata, D., Lingg, C.: Ankylosing spondylitis and spondylitis accompanying ulcerative colitis, regional enteritis, psoriasis and Reiter's disease. Arthr. Rheum. **14**, 291 (1971)
239. McGill, I.G.: An unusual neurological syndrome associated with ankylosing spondylitis. Guy's Hosp. Rep. **115**, 33–36 (1966)
240. McGregor, M.: The signifiance of certain

measurements of the skull in the diagnosis of basilar impression. Brit. J. Radiol. **21**, 171 (1948)
241. McRae, D.L.: Bony abnormalities in the region of the foramen magnum. Correlation of the anatomy and neurologic findings. Acta radiol. (Stockh.) **40**, 335–355 (1953)
242. McRae, D.L.: The significance of abnormalities of cervical spine. Amer. J. Roentgenol. **84**, 3 (1960)
243. Meijers, K.A.E.: Rheumatoid arthritis in the cervical spine. Acta orthop. belg. **38**, 33–37 (1972)
244. Meijers, K.A.E., Heerma van Voss, S.F.C., François, M.J.: Radiological changes in the cervical spine in ankylosing spondylitis. Ann. rheum. Dis. **27**, 333–338 (1968)
245. Meijers, K.A.E., Van Beusekom, G.T., Duyfjes, F., Luyendijk, N.: Treatment of dislocations in the cervical spine in rheumatoid arthritis and ankylosing spondylitis complicated by signs of cord compression: a follow-up study. Ann. rheum. Dis. **32**, 88–89 (1973)
246. Meijers, K.A.E., Van Beusekom, G.T., Luyendijk, N., Duyfjes, F.: Dislocation of the cervical spine with cord compression in rheumatoid arthritis. J. Bone Jt Surg. **56B**, 558–680 (1974)
247. Meikle, J.A.E., Wilkinson, N.: Rheumatoid involvement of the cervical spine. Radiological assessment. Ann. rheum. Dis. **30**, 154–161 (1971)
248. Merle, P., Georget, A.M., Viallet, J.F.: Etude radiologique dynamique des rapports de l'atlas et de l'axis chez l'enfant. J. Radiol. Électrol. **51**, 373 (1970)
249. Meunier, P., Courpron, P., Edouard, C., Bernard, J., Bringuier, J., Vignon, G.: Physiological senile involution and pathological rarefaction of bone. Quantitative and comparative histological data. Clin. Endocr. Metabol. **2**, 239–256 (1973)
250. Mikkelsen, W.M., Duff, I.F., Robinson, M.D.: Unusual manifestations of rheumatoid nodules. J. Mich. med. Soc. **54**, 292 (1955)
251. Morrisson, R.J.G.: Ankylosing spondylitis. Proc. roy. Soc. Med. **48**, 204 (1955)
252. Mosekilde, E.: Reumatoid arthritis i columna cervicalis. Røntgenologisk belyst. Nord. Med. **84**, 1507 (1970)
253. Nagashima, G.: Cervical myelopathy due to ossification of the posterior longitudinal ligament. J. Neurosurg. **37**, 653–660 (1972)
254. Nakano, K.K.: The entrapment neuropathies of rheumatoid arthritis. In: Rheumatoid arthritis, The orthopedic clinics of North America, Vol. 6, No. 3, pp. 837–860. Philadelphia: W.B. Saunders 1975
255. Nakano, K.K.: Neurologic complications of rheumatoid arthritis. In: Rheumatoid arthritis, The orthopedic clinics of North America, Vol. 6, No. 3, pp. 861–880. Philadelphia: W.B. Saunders 1975
256. Nathan, F.F., Bickel, W.H.: Spontaneous axial subluxation in a child as the first sign of juvenile rheumatoid arthritis. J. Bone Jt Surg. **50A**, 1675–1678 (1968)
257. Newman, P., Sweetnam, R.: Occipito-axial fusion. An operative technique and its indications. J. Bone Jt Surg. **51B**, 423–431 (1969)
258. Nordquist, L.: The sagittal diameter of the spinal cord and subarachnoid space in different age groups. Acta radiol. scand., Suppl. **227** (1964)
259. Onji, Y., Akiyama, H., Smimonura, Y., Ono, K., Ukuda, S., Mizuno, S.: Posterior paravertebral ossification causing cervical myelopathy. A report of 18 cases. J. Bone Jt Surg. **49A**, 1314–1328 (1967)
260. Ornilla Arota, E.: Afectation cervical en la artritis rhumatoidea. Rev. esp. Reum. **17**, 149–161 (1974)
261. Ornilla, E., Ansell, B.N., Swannella, J.: Cervical spine involvement in patients with chronic arthritis undergoing orthopaedic surgery. Ann. rheum. Dis. **31**, 364–368 (1972)
262. Ott, H., Wettstein, P., Mosimann, U.: Aspects radiologiques de la colonne cervicale dans l'arthrite rhumatoïde. Schweiz. med. Wschr. **100**, 1726–1730 (1970)
263. Ott, V.R., Wurm, M.: Spondylitis ankylopoetica. Darmstadt: Steinkopff 1957
264. Otto, W.: Zur Röntgenfunktions-Diagnostik der Halswirbelsäule in der Praxis. Fortschr. Röntgenstr. **83**, 834 (1955)
265. Paillast, J.E., Sedan, R.: Fracture et luxation du rachis cervical. J. Chir. **77**, 50–66 (1959)
266. Park, W.M., O'Brien, W.: Computer

assisted analysis of radiographic neck lesions in chronic rheumatoid arthritis. Acta radiol. [Diagn.] (Stockh.) **8**, 529–534 (1969)
267. Park, W.M., O'Brien, W.O.: Neck involvement in chronic rheumatoid arthritis, pp. 82–84. Symposium Ossium, London: E. & S. Livingstone 1970
268. Patte, D.: Arthrodèse cervico-occipitale. Rev. Chir. orthop. **55**, 675–681 (1969)
269. Pearson, C.M., Barnett, E., Kroening, R., Marmor, L., Murray, J.F., Peter, J.B., Salick, A.: Rheumatoid arthritis and its systemic manifestations. Ann. intern. Med. **65**, 1101–1130 (1966)
270. Penning, L.: Functional pathology of the cervical spine, p. 196. Amsterdam: Excerpta Medica Foundation 1968
271. Perovic, M.N., Kopits, S.E., Thompson, R.C.: Radiological evaluation of the spinal cord in congenital atlanto-axial dislocation. Radiology **109**, 713–719 (1973)
272. Peter, E., Schuler, B., Dihlmann, W.: Veränderungen der Wirbeldornfortsätze bei Arthritis mutilans. Dtsch. med. Wschr. **89**, 1990–1993 (1964)
273. Petersen, D.: Der rheumatische Schiefhals. Z. Orthop. **95**, 99–101 (1961)
274. Peterson, C.C., Jr., Silbinger, M.L.: Reiter's syndrome and psoriatic arthritis: their roentgen spectra and some interesting similarities. Amer. J. Roentgenol. **101**, 860–871 (1967)
275. Poirier, P., Charpy, A., Nicolas, A.: Traité d'anatomie humaine, Vol. 1. Paris: Masson et Cie. 1926
276. Potter, T.A., Barkins, R., Stillmann, J.S.: Occurrence of spondylitis in juvenile rheumatoid arthritis. Ann. rheum. Dis. **13**, 364–365 (1954)
277. Pratt, T.L.: Spontaneous dislocation of atlanto-axial articulation occurring in ankylosing spondylitis and rheumatoid arthritis. J. Fac. Radiol. (Lond.) **10**, 40–43 (1959)
278. Purser, D.W., Sharp, J.: Spontaneous atlanto-axial dislocation, complication of spondylitis. J. Bone Jt Surg. **39B**, 582 (1957)
279. Putz, R., Pomaroli, A.: Form und Funktion der Articulation atlanto-axialis lateralis. Acta anat. (Basel) **83**, 333–345 (1972)
280. Quyang, R., Mitchell, D.M., Rozdilsky, B.: Central nervous system involvement in rheumatoid disease. Neurology (Minneap.) **17**, 1099–1105 (1967)
281. Ramadier, J.O., Bombart, M.: Fracture et luxation du rachis cervical sans lésion médullaire. 1ère partie: Généralités. Lésions des deux premières vertèbres. 52 cas. Rev. Chir. orthop. **49**, 741–766 (1963)
282. Rana, N.A., Hancock, D.O., Taylor, A.R., Hill, A.G.S.: Atlanto-axial subluxation in rheumatoid arthritis. J. Bone Jt Surg. **55B**, 458–470 (1973)
283. Rana, N.A., Hancock, D.O., Taylor, A.R., Hill, A.G.S.: Upward translocation of the dens in rheumatoid arthritis. J. Bone Jt Surg. **55B**, 471–477 (1973)
284. Rana, N.A., Taylor, A.R.: Upward migration of the odontoid peg in rheumatoid arthritis. Proc. roy. Soc. Med. **64**, 717–718 (1971)
285. Rand, C.W.: The neurosurgical patient: his problems of diagnosis and care, p. 47. Springfield: Charles C. Thomas 1944
286. Ravault, P.P., Lejeune, E., Bouvier, M., Bochu, M., Jeanneret, J., Queneau, P., Fischer, L., Patricot, L.M., Cibert, M.: Luxations atloïdo-axoïdiennes au cours de la spondylarthrite ankylosante (à propos de 3 cas). J. Radiol. Électrol. **51**, 188–189 (1970)
287. Reid, J.D.: Effects of flexion-extension movements of head and spine upon spinal chord and nerve roots. J. Neurol. Neurosurg. Psychiat. **23**, 214 (1960)
288. Reinhardt, K.: Der Processus paracondylicus, paramastoideus, paraoccipitalis und der Processus supratransversarius des Atlas. Fortschr. Röntgenstr. **102**, 507 (1965)
289. Reitan, H.: Anterior subluxation of the atlas in rheumatic diseases. Acta rheum. scand. **14**, 24–34 (1968)
290. Rheumatoid cervical luxation. Brit. med. J. **1973**, 759–760
291. Robin de Andrade, J., Macnab, I.: Anterior occipitocervical fusion in rheumatoid arthritis. Arthr. Rheum. **12**, 423–426 (1969)
292. Robinson, H.S.: Rheumatoid arthritis. Atlanto-axial subluxation and its clinical presentation. J. Canad. Physiother. Ass. **18**, 206–216 (1966)
293. Rogers, L.: Spontaneous atlanto-axial dislocation. Pathogeny and treatment with

report of a new operative procedure. Brit. J. Surg. **49**, 63–65 (1961)
294. Rogers, W.A.: Fracture dislocation of the cervical spine. An end result study. J. Bone Jt Surg. **39A**, 341–376 (1957)
295. Rose, B.: L'arthrodèse cervico-occipitale. Thèse Paris 1968
296. Rössler, G., Schmeisser, A.: Die altersabhängige Beweglichkeitsminderung der Halswirbelsäule. Z. Alternsforsch. **11**, 75 (1957/1958)
297. Rotes-Querol, J.: La region cervical en los reumatismos inflamatorios: espondiloartritis anquilosante y poliartritis cronica. Rev. esp. Reum. **6**, 630–633 (1956)
298. Rouvière, H., Cordier, G., Delmas, A.: Anatomie humaine descriptive et topographique. 9th ed., Vol. 1. Paris: Masson 1962
299. Roy-Camille, R., Saillant, G.: Chirurgie du rachis cervical. Ostéosynthèse du rachis cervical supérieur. Nouv. Presse méd. 2847 2849 (1972)
300. Russel, M.L., Gordon, D.A., Coryzlo, M.A., McPherdan, R.S.: The cauda equina syndrome of ankylosing spondylitis. Ann. intern. Med. **78**, 551–554 (1973)
301. Saban, R.: Quest-ce que le proatlas? Ouest méd. **25**, 1391–1424 (1972)
302. Saffouri, M.H., Ward, P.H.: Surgical correction of dysphagia due to cervical osteophytes. Ann. Otol. (St. Louis) **83**, 65–70 (1974)
303. Sasaki, S.: Fatal basilar compression in arthritis mutilans: report of an unusual case. XIe Congrès Int. Mal. Rhumatismales, Mar del Plata, Buenos Aires, Yuste Publicidad, No. 265, 257–258 (1965)
304. Sawmiller, S.R., Wilde, A.M.: Spontaneous subluxation of the first and second cervical vertebrae in rheumatoid arthritis treated with spinal fusion: report of two cases. Cleveland Clin. Quart. **37**, 81–89 (1970)
305. Schilling, F.: Die Affektion der oberen Halswirbelsäule bei der Spondylitis ankylopoetica. Z. Rheumaforsch. **22**, 342–348 (1963)
306. Schilling, F.: Die bei chronischen rheumatischen Erkrankungen mögliche Beteiligung des Nervensystems: Polyneuropathie, periphere und medulläre Kompressionsyndrome. Therapiewoche **24**, 2950–2955 (1974)
307. Schilling, F.: Spondylite cervicale rhumatoïde. Rev. Rhum. **42**, 366–367 (1975)
308. Schilling, F., Haas, J.P., Schacherl, M.: Die spontane atlanto-axiale Dislokation (Ventralluxation des Atlas) bei chronischer Polyarthritis und Spondylitis ankylopoetica. Fortschr. Röntgenstr. **99**, 518–538 (1963)
309. Schilling, F., Schacherl, M.: Wirbelverschiebung und Blockwirbelbildung im Bereich der Halswirbelsäule auf rheumatisch-entzündlicher Grundlage. In: Möglichkeiten und Grenzen in der Röntgendiagnostik der Wirbelsäule, pp. 111–116. Stuttgart: Hippokrates 1964
310. Schilling, F., Schacherl, M., Bopp, A., Gamp, A., Haas, J.P.: Veränderungen der Halswirbelsäule (Spondylitis cervicalis) bei der chronischen rheumatischen Polyarthritis und bei der Spondylitis ankylopoetica. Radiologe **3**, 483–501 (1963)
311. Schmidt, H., Fischer, H.: Die okzipitale Dysplasie, pp. 69. Stuttgart: Thieme 1955
312. Scholz, V., Munchow, M.: Atlanto-axial Ventraldislokation im Kindesalter bei primär chronischer Polyarthritis. Kinderärztl. Prax. **41**, 31–42 (1973)
313. Seanan, W.B., Wells, J.: Destructive lesions of vertebral bodies in rheumatoid arthritis. Amer. J. Roentgenol. **86**, 241–250 (1961)
314. Serre, M., Betoulières, P., Simon, L., Janicot, J.Y., Lévy, F.: La charnière cervico-occipitale au cours de la polyarthrite chronique rhumatismale. A propos de 60 cas explorés. J. Radiol. Électrol. **45**, 361–363 (1964)
315. Serre, M., Rabischong, F., Simon, L., Jambon, P.: Etude anatomique d'une charnière cervico-occipitale au cours d'une polyarthrite chronique rhumatismale. Rev. Rhum. **30**, 648–650 (1963)
316. Serre, M., Simon, L., Janicot, J.Y., Levy, F.: Les affections rhumatismales de la charnière cervico-occipitale. Rev. Rhum. **30**, 518–544 (1963)
317. Serre, M., Simon, L., Janicot, J.Y., Levy, F.: La luxation atloïdo-axoïdienne. Complication fréquente de la polyarthrite chronique rhumatismale. Presse méd. **72**, 213–219 (1964)

318. Sèze, S. de, Djian, A., Abdelmoula, J.: Etude radiologique de la dynamique dans le plan sagittal. Une contribution radiophysiologique à l'étude pathogénique des arthroses cervicales. Rev. Rhum. **18**, 111–116 (1951)
319. Sèze, S. de, Djian, A., Caroit, M.: Luxation atloïdo-axoïdienne d'origine rhumatismale. Rev. Rhum. **24**, 192–199 (1957)
320. Sèze, S. de, Djian, A., Debeyre, N.: Luxations atloïdo-axoïdiennes au cours de la polyarthrite rhumatoïde. Leur fréquence. Intérêt des épreuves radiodynamiques pour leur dépistage. A propos de 10 observations personnelles découvertes au cours d'une enquête portant sur 103 polyarthrites. Rev. Rhum. **30**, 560–565 (1963)
321. Sèze, S. de, Djian, A., Martin, M.: De l'utilité des épreuves radiologiques fonctionnelles dans les traumatismes cervicaux (atlas-axis). Rev. Rhum. **18**, 318–384 (1951)
322. Sèze, S. de, Jurmand, S.M., Levernieux, J., Durieu, J., Gueguen, Y., Hubault, A.: A propos de 7 cas de luxation cervicale. Evolution, clinique et traitement. Rev. Rhum. **19**, 239–244 (1952)
323. Sharp, J.: Cervical spine. In: Radiological aspects of rheumatoid arthritis. Proceedings of an international Symposium, Excerpta Medica International Congress Serie, No. 61, pp. 219–231 (1964)
324. Sharp, J., Purser, D.W.: Spontaneous atlanto-axial dislocation in ankylosing spondylitis and rheumatoid arthritis. Ann. rheum. Dis. **20**, 47–77 (1961)
325. Sharp, J., Purser, D.W., Lawrence, J.S.: Rheumatoid arthritis of cervical spine in adult. Ann. rheum. Dis. **17**, 303–313 (1958)
326. Sholkoff, S.D., Glickman, M.G., Steinbach, M.L.: Roentgenology of Reiter's syndrome. Radiology **97**, 497 (1970)
327. Siaud, J.R., Auquier, L.: Les myélopathies par atteinte rhumatoïde du rachis cervical. Rhumatologie **27**, 385–390 (1975)
328. Sicard, A.: Les séquelles des lésions traumatiques de la charnière cervico-occipitale. Rev. Rhum. **30**, 545–551 (1963)
329. Sievers, K., Nissila, M., Sievers, V.N.: Cerebral vasculitis visualized by angiography in juvenile rheumatoid arthritis simulating brain tumor. Acta rheum. scand. **14**, 222–232 (1968)
330. Simon, L., Allieu, Y., Sany, J., Blotman, F., Claustre, J.: Polyarthrite rhumatoïde de l'adulte: rééducation, réadaptation. In: Encyclopédie Médico-Chirurgicale: Kinésithérapie-Rééducation fonctionnelle, Paris, 1975, 4.0.02, 26290, A 10, pp. 1–28
331. Smillowicz, M.: Atlanto-axial subluxation with paresis of the extremities in the course of rheumatoid arthritis. Rheumatologia **8**, 341–346 (1970)
332. Smith, P.H., Benn, R.T., Sharp, J.: Natural history of rheumatoid cervical luxations. Ann. rheum. Dis. **31**, 431–439 (1972)
333. Stammers, F.A.R., Frazer, P.: Spontaneous dislocation of the atlas with report of a case. Lancet **1933II**, 1203–1205
334. Steinbach, H.L., Jensen, P.L.: Roentgenographic changes in the arthritides (Part II). Seminars in Arthritis and Rheumatism **5**, 203–246 (1976)
335. Steiner, J.W., Geldbloon, A.J.: Intracranial manifestations in two cases of systemic rheumatoid disease. Arthr. Rheum. **2**, 537–547 (1959)
336. Stevens, J.C., Cartlidge, N.E.F., Saunders, M., Appeley, A., Hall, M., Shaw, D.A.: Atlanto-axial subluxation and cervical myelopathy in rheumatoid arthritis. Quart. J. Med. **40**, 391–408 (1971)
337. Still, G.F.: New chronic joint disease in children. Brit. med. J. **1896II**
338. Stoia, J.: Die Wirbelsäule bei primär chronischer Polyarthritis im Kindesalter. Z. Rheumaforsch. **22**, 187–192 (1963)
339. Storey, G.: Changes on the cervical spine in rheumatoid arthritis with compression of the cord. Ann. phys. Med. **4**, 216–218 (1958)
340. Storig, E., Schilling, F.: Zur spontanen atlanto-axialen Dislokation. Z. Orthop. **97**, 231–234 (1963)
341. Storig, E., Schilling, F.: Die Fraktur der Halswirbelsäule bei Spondylarthitis ankylopoetica. Z. Orthop. **97**, 492–502 (1963)
342. Stratford, J.: Myelopathy caused by atlanto-axial dislocation. J. Neurosurg. **14**, 97–100 (1957)
343. Streda, A.: Ankylosis of cervical spine in the adult age as a manifestation of juvenile rheumatoid arthritis. Fysiat. Rheumatol. Vestn. **52**, 276–278 (1974)
344. Sullivan, A.W.: Subluxation of atlanto-ax-

ial joint: Sequel to inflammatory processes of neck. J. Radiat. **35**, 451 (1949)

345. Sullivan, C.R., Bruwer, A.J., Harris, L.E.: Hypermobility of the cervical spine in children: A pitfall in the diagnosis of cervical dislocation. Amer. Surg. **95**, 636 (1958)
346. Sukoff, M.H., Kadin, M.M., Moran, T.: Transoral decompression for myelopathy caused by rheumatoid arthritis of the cervical spine. Case report. J. Neurosurg. **37**, 493–497 (1974)
347. Swanberg, H.: Anterior dislocation of the atlas following tonsillectomy. J. Amer. med. Ass. **72**, 107–108 (1919)
348. Sweetnam, E.: Atlanto-axial instability in rheumatoid arthritis. Ann. rheum. Dis. **29**, 333–335 (1972)
349. Swinson, D.R., Hamilton, E.D., Mathews, J.A., Yates, D.A.H.: Vertical subluxation of the axis in rheumatoid arthritis. Ann. rheum. Dis. **31**, 359–363 (1972)
350. Teboul, A.: L'impression basilaire au cours de la polyarthrite rhumatoïde. Mémoire C.E.S. Rhumatologie, Paris, 1967, p. 104
351. Tedesco, B., Grisel, P., Desfosses, P., Tassin, J.: Deux nouveaux cas d'énucléation de l'atlas par torticolis naso-pharyngien. Bull. Soc. Pediat. Paris **18**, 252–262 (1930)
352. Teissier: Les luxations atloïdo-axoïdiennes. Thèse Paris, 1841
353. Testut, L., Latarjet, A.: Traité d'anatomie humaine, 9th ed., Vol. 1. Paris: G. Doin 1948
354. Thalmann, M., Scholl, M., Tonz, O.: Spontane Atlasdislokation bei einem Kind mit Trisomie 21 und rheumatoider Arthritis. Helv. paediat. Acta **27**, 391–403 (1972)
355. Theron, J., Djindjian, R.: Technique de phlébographie rachidienne cervicale par cathétérisme. J. Radiol. Électrol. **54**, 105–111 (1973)
356. Thiebaut, F., Wackenheim, A., Vrousos, C.: Un nouveau repère pour le diagnostic radiologique des déplacements de la dent de l'axis dans les traumatismes et les malformations de la charnière cervico-occipitale. Rev. Oto-neuro-Ophtal. **32**, 410 (1960)
357. Thomas, W.H.: Surgical management of the rheumatoid cervical spine. In: Rheumatoid arthritis. The orthopedic clinics of North America, Vol. 6, No. 5, pp. 793–800. Philadelphia: W.B. Saunders 1975
358. Thompson, H.: The "Hals" traction apparatus. A method of external splinting of the cervical spine after injury. J. Bone Jt Surg. **44B**, 655–661 (1962)
359. Thompson, H.: Transoral fusion of the upper cervical spine. Proc. roy. Soc. Med. **63**, 893–898 (1970)
360. Titrud, L.A., McKinlay, C.A., Camp, W.E., Hannah, R.B.: Non traumatic atlanto-axial dislocation. Report of a case with recovery after quadriplegia. J. Neurosurg. **6**, 174–177 (1949)
361. Torklus, D. von, Gehle, W.: Die obere Halswirbelsäule, p. 106. Stuttgart: Thieme 1970
362. Trolard, D.: Les articulations de la tête avec la colonne vertébrale. J. Anat. (Paris) **33**, 105–128 (1897)
363. Van Beusekom, G.T.: The neurological syndrome associated with cervical luxation in rheumatoid arthritis. Acta orthop. belg. **38**, 38–39 (1972)
364. Van der Meer, P.: Rheumatoid arthritis and cervical spine. Acta rheum. scand. **11**, 81–96 (1965)
365. Van Kerckhove, H.: Involvement of the lateral atlanto-axial joints as first and late symptom of rheumatoid arthritis. Acta rheum. scand. **16**, 197–210 (1970)
366. Vaughan, B.: Lateral tomography of atlanto-axial joint in rheumatoid disease. Aust. Radiol. **12**, 58–60 (1968)
367. Verhaeghe, A., Lesage, R., Delcambre, B., Gosselin, B.: Spondylodiscites chroniques au cours de la polyarthrite rhumatoïde. Rev. Rhum. **36**, 124–130 (1969)
368. Verjaal, A., Hardner, N.C.: Backward luxation of the atlas. Acta radiol. [Diagn.[(Stockh.) **3**, 173–176 (1965)
369. Vicas, E.B.: Fractures de la colonne cervicale ankylosée par la maladie de Marie-Strumpell. Un. méd. Can. **101**, 1818–1821 (1972)
370. Vignon, G., Bied, J.C.: Rôle de la corticothérapie dans l'ostéoporose vertébrale de la polyarthrite rhumatoïde. Rev. Rhum. **35**, 87–89 (1968)
371. Vignon, G., Cibert, M., Minaire, P.: Les luxations atloïdo-axoïdiennes des rhumatismes inflammatoires chroniques. Ann. Méd. phys. **16**, 226–234 (1973)

372. Vignon, G., Pansu, D., Bied, J.C.: L'ostéoporose de la polyarthrite rhumatoïde. Rev. Rhum. **34**, 235–242 (1967)
373. Vignon, G., Patet, R.: La luxation antérieure spontanée de l'atlas (à propos d'un cas observé dans une polyarthrite rhumatoïde). Rev. lyon. Méd. **4**, 693–702 (1955)
374. Vlahovitch, B., Fuentes, J.M.: Traitement chirurgical des métastases du rachis cervical. Principales orientations. Nouv. Presse méd. **4**, 2493–2497 (1975)
375. Voluter, G., Werner, A.: Luxation atloïdo-axoïdienne antérieure non traumatique chez l'adulte. J. Radiol. Électrol. **37**, 176–178 (1956)
376. Wackenheim, A.: Rhumatismes cervico-occipitaux. France méd. **30**, 429–434 (1967)
377. Wackenheim, A.: Problèmes radiographiques pour l'étude rhumatologique de la charnière cervico-occipitale. J. Radiol. Électrol. **49**, 215–225 (1968)
378. Wackenheim, A.: Diagnostic radiologique des formes congénitales, des formes intermittentes et des formes progressives de sténose du canal rachidien au niveau de l'atlas. Acta radiol. (Stockh.) **9**, 759–768 (1969)
379. Wackenheim, A.: Le bloc fonctionnel occipito-atloïdien. J. Radiol. Électrol. **54**, 401–402 (1973)
380. Wackenheim, A.: Roentgen diagnosis of the cranio-vertebral region. Berlin-Heidelberg-New York: Springer 1974
381. Wackenheim, A.: Une méthode de notation de l'épreuve radiodynamique de flexion-extension cervicale. J. méd. Strasbourg **6**, 25–29 (1975)
382. Wackenheim, A., Babin, E., Thiebaut, M.S.D., Lopez, F.: Une nouvelle épreuve fonctionnelle pour l'exploration de la dynamique cervico-occipitale. Le glissement de la tête vers l'avant et vers l'arrière. Concours méd. **91**, 7130–7136 (1969)
383. Wackenheim, A., Bourjat, P.: La dislocation odonto-atloïdienne antéro-postérieure d'origine rhumatismale. Rev. Oto-neuro-ophtal. **40**, 212–216 (1960)
383a. Wackenheim, A., Braun, J.P.: Roentgendiagnosis of the veins of the posterior fossa. Berlin-Heidelberg-New York: Springer 1977 (to be published)
384. Wackenheim, A., Dirheimer, Y.: Les formes cervicales de l'hyperostose vertébrale. Sem. Hôp. Paris **46**, 2743–2749 (1970)
385. Wackenheim, A., Dirheimer, Y.: Diagnostic radiologique des localisations rhumatismales au niveau de la charnière cervico-occipitale. Paris: Société Française de Radiologie Médicale 1974 (with 35 slides)
386. Wackenheim, A., Dirheimer, Y., Dries, G.: Un appareil d'immobilisation sélective du rachis cervical. J. méd. Strasbourg **5**, 215–218 (1974)
387. Walcher, K., Hohmann, D., Gruska, M.: Röntgenologisch funktionelle Studien bei der Spondylitis cervicalis rheumatica. Z. Orthop. **105**, 316–333 (1958)
388. Watson-Jones, R.: Spontaneous hyperaemic dislocation of the atlas. Proc. roy. Soc. Med. **25**, 586–590 (1932)
389. Wayne, J.E.: Fracture-dislocation of the cervical part of the spine column in patients with ankylosing spondylitis. Mayo Clin. Proc. **43**, 714–721 (1968)
390. Webb, F.W.S., Mickmann, J.A., Brew, D.S.J.: Death from vertebral artery thrombosis in rheumatoid arthritis. Brit. med. J. **1968II**, 537–588
391. Weigl, E., Wruck, E.: Veränderungen der Halswirbelsäule bei der rheumatoiden Arthritis. Radiol. diagn. (Berl.) **10**, 655–660 (1969)
392. Weiss, L.A., Freemafer, A.A.: Atraumatic subluxation and dislocation of the cervical spine in rheumatoid arthritis. Clin. Orthop. **34**, 53 (1964)
393. Weissmann, N.W., Sosman, J.L.: The radiology of rheumatoid arthritis. In: Rheumatoid arthritis. The orthopedic clinics of North America, Vol. 6, No. 3, pp. 653–674. Philadelphia: W.B. Saunders 1975
394. Went, H.: Zur Manifestation eines Proatlas. Fortschr. Röntgenstr. **95**, 370 (1962)
395. Werne, S.: Spontaneous dislocation of the atlas (as a complication in rheumatoid arthritis). Acta rheum. scand. **3**, 101–107 (1957)
396. Werne, S.: Studies in spontaneous atlas dislocation. Acta orthop. scand., Suppl. **23** (1957)
397. Werne, S.: Über normale Atlasbewegungen und Atlasfehlstellungen. Z. Orthop. **93**, 205 (1960)
398. Werner, A.: La luxation atloïdo-axo-

idienne de l'adulte. Techniques de réduction et d'ostéosynthèse. Neurochirurgie **6**, 205–215 (1960)

399. Whaley, K., Dick, W.C.: Fatal subaxial dislocation of cervical spine in rheumatoid arthritis. Brit. med. J. **1968 II**, 31
400. Wilkinson, M., Bywaters, E.G.L.: Clinical fractures and course of ankylosing spondylitis. As seen in a follow-up of 222 Hospital referred cases. Ann. rheum. Dis. **17**, 209–228 (1958)
401. Williams, L.E., Bland, J.M., Lipson, R.L.: Cervical spine subluxation and massive osteolysis in the upper extremities in rheumatoid arthritis. Arthr. Rheum. **9**, 348–360 (1966)
402. Wittek, A.: Ein Fall von Distensionsluxation im Atlanto-epistropheal-Gelenk. Münch. med. Wschr. **35**, 1836–1837 (1908)
403. Wollin, D.G., Botterell, E.M.: Symmetrical forward luxation of the atlas. Amer. J. Roentgenol. **79**, 575 (1958)
404. Woodruff, F.P., Dewing, S.B.: Fracture of the cervical spine in patients with ankylosing spondylitis. Radiology **80**, 17–21 (1963)
405. Wosko, I.: Atlanto-axoid subluxation in progressive rheumatism. Chir. Narząd. Ruchu. **28**, 747–749 (1963)
406. Zeidler, H., Wittenborg, A., Vogelsang, M., Weidner, A., Kahlstorf, J.: Neurologische Komplikationen bei chronischer Polyarthritis der Halswirbelsäule. Dtsch. med. Wschr. **98**, 988–992 (1973)
407. Ziff, M., Contreras, V., McEven, C.: Spondylitis in post-pubertal patients with rheumatoid arthritis of juvenile onset. Ann. rheum. Dis. **15**, 40–45 (1956)

Subject Index

Axial and axoid are strictly synonymous terms which are used in the text, but only the term "axial" is entered into the subject index.

Springer-Verlag
Berlin
Heidelberg
New York

H.G. FASSBENDER

Pathology of Rheumatic Diseases

Translated from the German Edition by G. Loewi

444 figures. XI, 353 pages. 1975.
ISBN 3-540-07289-6
Distribution rights for Japan: Igaku Shoin Ltd., Tokyo

Contents: History of the Rheumatic Diseases. – Components of Connective Tissue. – Reactions. – Rheumatic Fever. – Rheumatoid Arthritis. – Juvenile Rheumatoid Arthritis and Still's Disease. – Sjögren's Syndrome. – Ankylosing Spondylitis. – Psoriatic Arthritis. – Gout. – Chondrocalcinosis. – Osteo-Arthritis. – Non-Articular Rheumatism. – Experimental Arthritis. – References. – Subject Index.

During the past decades our knowledge both of the rheumatic diseases and of clinical and experimental immunology expanded enormously. Therefore, in a comprehensive discussion of the pathogenetic mechanisms and underlying morphology the author presents many new findings relating to rheumatic disease, including rheumatic fever, chronic polyarthritis, ankylosing spondylitis, psoriatic arthritis, gout, rheumatoid arthritis, and fibrositis. He pays particular attention to the dynamics of pathological processes and the way they find expression in the clinical symptoms of the disease. To aid the reader in understanding the complex relationships now known to exist in rheumatic disease, the text is supported by many histological and radiological illustrations, and light, electron and scanning-electron micrographs. Presented in this way, the pathogenetic mechanisms offer clues to the form of treatment to be given.

Bayer – Symposium 6

Experimental Models of Chronic Inflammatory Diseases

Editors: L.E. Glynn, H.D. Schlumberger

142 figures. 62 tables. XIV, 460 pages. 1977.
ISBN 3-540-08095-3
(Bayer Symposium VI held at Grosse Ledder near Cologne, Germany, May 20–22, 1976)

Contents: Experimental Models of Rheumatoid Lesions. – Experimental Models and Systemic Lupus. – Recent Approaches to Experimental Immune Complex Disease and Allergic Vasculitis. – Arthritis During the Course of Experimental of Natural Infection. – Control Mechanisms in Inflammatory Responses. – Should we Stimulate or Suppress the Inflammatory Response?

The Proceedings of the Sixth Bayer Symposium are devoted to the discussion and interpretation of experimental models of chronic inflammatory diseases. The different sections deal with experimental models of rheumatoid lesions, experimental models of systemic lupus erythematosus, recent approaches to experimental immunocomplex disease and allergic vasculitis, and arthritis during the course of experimental or natural infection. The final session is directed to the question: "Should we stimulate or suppress the inflammatory response?"

Since the etiology and pathogenesis of chronic inflammatory diseases in humans are largely unknown, the experimental models of such diseases or features of these diseases need thorough interpretation as to their relevance to human disease. The Proceedings of this Bayer Symposium will contribute to a better understanding and evaluation of models of chronic inflammatory diseases which are the most important prerequisites for new therapeutic approaches to progressive inflammatory diseases in man.

Advances in Neurosurgery
Volume 4

Lumbar Disc
Adult Hydrocephalus

Proceedings of the 27th Annual Meeting of the „Deutsche Gesellschaft für Neurochirurgie", Berlin, September 12–15, 1976
Editors: R. Wüllenweber, M. Brock, J. Hamer, M. Klinger, O. Spoerri

154 figures, 67 tables. XXII, 338 pages (12 pages in German). 1977.
ISBN 3-540-08100-3
Distribution rights for Japan: Nankodo Co. Ltd. Tokyo

Contents: Lumbar Disc. – Adult Hydrocephalus. – Free Communications.

Volume 4 of *Advances in Neurosurgery* is dedicated to two subjects which constitute a daily challenge to the neurosurgeon.

The first part of this volume deals with the *Lumbar Disc*. Special consideration was given to the problems of recurrences and of disc hernation in youngsters and elderly patients. Prognostic and catamnestic aspects have been evaluated through an extensive joint statistic inquiry.

In the second part, attention is focused on *Adult Hydrocephalus*. The various diagnostic procedures presently employed – including those of nuclear medicine – are analyzed as concerns their significance for therapy and prognosis. The clinical applications of continuous intracranial pressure monitoring, and the pathophysiologic importance of the obtained data are discussed.

The third part of this volume contains a series of contributions on neurotraumatology (head injuries, brain edema, intensive care) and on neurophysiological topics.

Advances and Technical Standards in Neurosurgery

Editors: H. Krayenbühl (Managing Editor), J. Brihaye, F. Loew, V. Logue, S. Mingrino, B. Pertuiset, L. Symon, H. Troupp, M.G. Yasargil

Vol. 4

66 figures. Approx. 170 pages. 1977.
ISBN 3-211-81423-X

Contents: N.A. Lassen, D.H. Ingvar: Clinical Relevance of Cerebral Blood Flow Measurements. – G.W. Taylor, J.S.P. Lumley: Extra-Cranial Surgery for Cerebrovascular Disease. – J. Retif: Intrathecal Injection of a Neurolytic Solution for the Relief of Intractable Pain. – L. Symon: Olfactory Groove and Suprasellar Moningicmas. – M.G. Yasargil, R.D. Smith, J.C. Gasser: Microsurgical Approach to Acoustic Neurinomas. – G. Debrun, P. Lacour, J.P. Caron: Balloon Arterial Catheter Techniques in the Treatment of Arterial Intracranial Diseases.

Springer-Verlag
Berlin
Heidelberg
New York

GPSR Compliance
The European Union's (EU) General Product Safety Regulation (GPSR) is a set of rules that requires consumer products to be safe and our obligations to ensure this.

If you have any concerns about our products, you can contact us on

ProductSafety@springernature.com

In case Publisher is established outside the EU, the EU authorized representative is:

Springer Nature Customer Service Center GmbH
Europaplatz 3
69115 Heidelberg, Germany

www.ingramcontent.com/pod-product-compliance
Lightning Source LLC
Chambersburg PA
CBHW061212240926
51846CB00006B/1193
* 9 7 8 3 6 4 2 6 6 6 0 7 0 *